ASTHMA HAY FEVER AND OTHER ALLERGIES

ASTHMA HAY FEVER AND OTHER ALLERGIES

and how to live with them

Elizabeth Forsythe

WILLIAM LUSCOMBE PUBLISHER LIMITED

First published in Great Britain by
William Luscombe Publisher Limited
The Mitchell Beazley Group
Artists House
14 Manette Street London W1V 5LB
1975

ISBN 0 86002 089 4 (cased)
0 86002 139 4 (paperback)

Text set in 12pt Photon Imprint, printed by photolithography,
and bound in Great Britain at The Pitman Press, Bath.

Contents

◆◇◆◇

1 What is allergy?

This sounds a very simple question to ask, and has probably been asked many times by some of the millions of sufferers of different types of allergy in the United Kingdom. It is, however, an extremely difficult question to answer because many of the details of the changes which take place in an allergic reaction are still being investigated. Here we will keep to fairly well established facts, and try to explain the whole problem in as straightforward a way as possible.

It is important that the problem of allergy should be widely understood because about 1 in 10 of the entire population of the United Kingdom suffers from one type of allergy or another. By and large it is fair to say that there is no real cure for allergy. Allergic conditions are ones that can often be helped medically, but in the long run have to be lived with. Therefore, anything which improves the understanding and tolerance of the patient for his problems will be a help, not just to a few, but to several millions.

Allergy can be defined as an altered response by somebody to an antigen. An antigen in a normal person is sometimes something, often a germ of some sort, which when it meets the body causes it to produce antibodies which deal with the invader. In allergy, the antigen may be something which is quite harmless to most people, such as house dust, but in the allergic person produces an allergic type of antibody which leads not to immunity, but to an allergic reaction.

Most people when they come into contact with an antigen such as a bacterium or virus resist the infection and produce antibodies to it. The infection can either be caught naturally as with mumps or measles, or can be given artificially by an injection of dead or weakened germs, as can be done with measles, whooping-cough, diphtheria and other immunisations. In either case, the body produces antibodies against the infection. In many illnesses and immunisations, the body keeps its resistance to a further infection by the same antigen indefinitely. Sometimes the resistance is only short-lived as with the common cold. In this way, the influx of an antigen on the body and production of an antibody is a good thing, and obviously one to be inherited with gratitude.

Most people do not produce any type of reaction or antibody when they come into contact with substances which are 'foreign' to their own body such as pollen or dander from an animal's coat. However, 1 in 10 people do react to these 'foreign' substances which may be described as allergic antigens or allergens. When they come into contact with one of these things to which their particular body is allergic, instead of producing a useful antibody, they produce an allergic antibody which is sometimes known as a reagin. This type of antibody, instead of being an asset, is always a nuisance, and can sometimes have very dire consequences as will be described later in this chapter.

People who have this type of allergic reaction are sometimes called atopic. The word atopy comes from the Greek word atopia which means unusualness. One has to remember that probably at least 5 million people in the United Kingdom alone suffer from this type of unusualness, so it is fairly normal to be unusual in this way.

It is widely agreed that one of the most important factors in the making of an atopic person is heredity. It is very difficult to understand why hereditary conditions which are apparently of no use and often of very definite harm to the individual should be so common. Many severe hereditary disorders tend to breed themselves out of the population because the sufferers may not survive long enough to breed. Allergy is very seldom life threatening, and therefore does not come into this category. With some inherited diseases there is a known pattern of inheritance, and the outcome for the children can be predicted. With allergies there is no such definite pattern, but there is no doubt at all about the familial incidence. A father may have hay fever and one of his children have eczema as a baby, and develop asthma as he grows older. If both parents have allergies there is very little more chance of the children being allergic than if only one parent has an allergy. Certainly, an allergy in one of the parents, even if severe, is no reason for not having children.

The allergen that sets off an allergic reaction may be pollen, or animal dander, house dust, mould spores, or one of many other things. It may be breathed in or swallowed in food as happens with such allergens as nuts, chocolates or fish. The thing that allergic people have in common, and it is probably the part that heredity plays, is that when they come into contact with one of these 'foreign' substances, instead of ignoring it, their bodies produce allergic antibody.

This might be described as a perverted way of producing useful immunity to something. Allergic antibody, or reagin, is the same type of substance as a useful antibody. It is an immunoglobulin, and is described as belonging to the IgE class. Instead of acting in any useful way, it becomes potentially destructive and disease producing, instead of disease resisting. The first time a potentially allergic person meets an antigen nothing happens. If he is to become sensitive to this antigen, reagin begins to form in his body. Reaginic or allergic antibody is probably made in the lymph nodes of the body, where other types of immunoglobulins, including useful antibodies are made, but this is not known for sure. Reaginic antibody has a special talent for fixing itself to the outside of certain cells found particularly in the mucous membranes of the body, and in the loose connective tissue just under the skin. Mucous membranes are all those warm, soft, moist areas which line the mouth, throat, lungs and gut, amongst other parts.

The cells that are caught up with reaginic antibody are called mask cells. These are closely related to one of the types of white cell found in the blood. These mask cells are invisible to the naked eye, and as well as having a nucleus, are packed with granules which take part in an allergic reaction.

When an allergic person meets an antigen, to which he is sensitive, for the second time, the allergic mechanism is all ready to have a go at his cost. The allergen, which it must be remembered is entirely harmless to 9 out of 10 of the population, sticks itself on to the outside of the mask cells in the areas where it comes into contact. This may be in a number of places, including the respiratory passages and the gut. The reaginic antibody is an immunoglobulin, and the allergic person always has an increased amount of this substance, IgE in his blood. The substance is, however, present in small quantities in the blood of normal people so that it cannot be entirely harmful.

When a mask cell has reaginic antibody on it and meets a particular allergen for the second time, a very dramatic reaction takes place. The cell breaks up, the granules are released, and they let loose a number of substances including histamine. Histamine probably produces most of the results of the common types of allergic reaction, but there are less common types of allergic reaction where histamine plays no part at all. Amongst the actions of histamine are the dilatation of the smallest blood vessels and capillaries. This causes swelling of the area. Histamine also increases the permeability of the capillaries, and fluid is poured out of them. It also causes the contraction of smooth muscle, muscle which is not under one's own control. This in part causes the wheezing in asthma, and the colic when there is allergy of the gut. The exact type of illness produced depends on the sensitivity of the person, and the part or parts where they are sensitive to particular allergens.

The amount of IgE in the person's body can be measured by very delicate tests with radio-isotopic substances. This is only done as part of research work and not in the routine tests for allergies. It is found that in allergic asthma the level is raised in 60% of people, and the average level is six times that of normal people. The level of IgE rises after a patient has been exposed to the allergen to which he is sensitive.

The type of reaction which has been described is sometimes medically called the Type 1 type of hypersensitivity. This accounts for most of the commonly met types of allergy, including eczema, some cases of asthma, allergic rhinitis which is a chronic allergy of the nose, and hay fever. The type of allergy produced will depend in part on the age of the sufferer, and on the route of entry of the allergen. In infants, the commonest types of allergy are of the gut, causing sometimes allergy to cow's milk, or to wheat containing cereal, and also eczema which may also be caused by food. Allergic reactions in infants seem to be on the increase, possibly due to more usual feeding with cow's milk instead of breast milk, and partly due to earlier starting of mixed feeding. In a few parts of the country there seems to be a slight swing back to breast feeding, but in most parts it is a lost cause. Later weaning is now advised for many reasons. One of the benefits of late weaning is delay in introducing foreign substances to the baby's gut which may act as allergens.

The babies of allergic parents who themselves have an allergic tendency will sooner or later meet an allergen to which they will produce an allergic antibody, and later an allergic reaction. It is obviously impossible to protect these growing children from every potential allergen. However, some protection can be given in the early months by breast feeding which is usually successful if the mother sees sufficiently good reasons for persevering. The delay in starting mixed feeding, particularly wheat cereal and egg white is also helpful in preventing the onset of an allergic reaction. By delaying the introduction of these substances in the blood, trouble may be avoided because the gut of the small infant is more easily penetrated by these things.

In hay fever, allergic rhinitis which is not connected with grass pollen, and often continuing throughout the year, most types of asthma and eczema, the reactions described above occur, and histamine is released from the mask cells in the mucous membranes or skin. This produces a local reaction like an inflammation but not caused by germs. The area becomes swollen, mucus or fluid is poured out, and in asthma and in allergy of the gut, smooth muscle contracts.

In hay fever the allergen is pollen, most commonly grass, but it can be the pollen of other flowers or of some trees. It does not usually start before the age of four years old. The pollen lands on the mucosal lining of the nose or the conjunctivae of the eyes, the reactions described take place, and histamine is released. This causes swelling of the mucosae, out-pouring of fluid, and a local irritation of the nose, eyes and often the throat. This type of reaction responds to the group of drugs known as antihistamines, and can usually be controlled by them. If hay fever is severe, and is not controlled, the allergic reaction can spread and the patient may develop asthma. These attacks occur most commonly at night.

In allergic rhinitis the same reaction takes place as described above, but there is no seasonal variation connected with pollen, and it may be present at any time of year. Allergic rhinitis may start at a younger age than hay fever, and sometimes accounts for the toddler who is said to have a perpetual cold.

Asthma is often caused in the same way. Blockage of the small tubes in the lung occurs by the swelling of the mucosae, out-pouring of mucus, and contraction of the smooth muscle.

Most of the types of allergy caused by rupture of the mask cells and the release of histamine and other substances, start fairly soon after exposure to the allergen, and clear up quickly with the appropriate treatment which will be described in Chapter 3, and in detail with the different allergies.

Type II reaction in medical terms, appears in rather a different way, and in some ways is the opposite of Type I. The antigen is stuck on to certain cells, often red blood cells in the body, the antibody is the invader and not the invaded. This happens when the wrong blood is given in a blood transfusion, and the red blood cells are destroyed.

There is another type of allergic reaction which is medically called Type III, or Arthus reaction. The antigen and the antibody react together in tissue spaces, and a precipitate is formed which can block small blood vessels. It takes several hours to start after exposure to the offending antigen, and lasts from 24 to 36 hours. The reaction may include a fever, pains in the muscles, aching and a rise in the number of white cells in the blood. All these suggest an infection rather than an allergy. This sort of reaction cannot be helped with antihistamines.

A reaction like this can cause what is called serum sickness. It used to occur after the injection of large amounts of horse serum in the treatment of diphtheria. Sometimes, as well as the fever and aches and pains, it caused skin rashes and affected the urine. Such reactions are rare now because diphtheria is prevented by immunisation rather than treated by horse serum.

Another way in which this type of reaction shows itself is in what is known as farmer's lung. IgE is not present in excess in this type of reaction, but there is an increase in other sorts of immunoglobulins. The disease is caused by a type of allergy to the spores in mouldy hay. The spores are very small and get into the tiniest passages in the lung. The disease is rather like asthma, but is often more difficult to treat and there are changes that can be seen in an X-ray.

When skin testing for allergens which cause asthma, a positive result is usually seen in about 20 minutes. However, in farmer's lung, the reaction takes 4 to 5 hours to appear. This will be described more fully in the next chapter.

Type IV reaction is the last known type of allergic reaction. It depends on certain sensitized white cells called mononuclears in the body. This type of reaction is probably responsible for contact dermatitis which is a type of skin disease caused by close contact with such irritant substances as dyes and some chemicals. It also may account for what is known as auto-immune diseases, and for the rejection of organ transplants such as heart and liver.

There are one or two ways in which acute types of allergy

can cause a medical emergency for which you need medical attention immediately. Anaphylactic shock is a state of shock which may be very serious. The patient feels very ill, is pale and sweating. The heart beat is rapid and he may feel very frightened. The cause of such violent reaction is most often the injection of a vaccine or a drug to which the patient has previously been sensitized. Of drugs, Penicillin is the most common culprit. If you are sensitive to Penicillin, you should always tell a new doctor or dentist who is treating you. This very alarming condition will be discussed more fully in chapter 12, on Drugs and Allergy.

Another type of acute allergic reaction is called angioneurotic oedema. This usually happens after eating of food to which the patient is sensitized. There is swelling of the lips and tongue, eyelids and face. The throat may also get swollen and cause difficulty in breathing. This alarming condition will be described more fully in Chapter 11 on the Gut and Allergy.

❖❖❖❖

There is no investigation more important when trying to solve the problems of an allergic illness, than for the doctor to get a good history. This means the doctor knows all the details of the trouble, and no further tests may be really necessary to solve the problem, although further tests are, in fact, usually done to make absolutely sure that the doctor's clinical judgement is right. A good account of the illness depends not only on the patience and the detective skill of the doctor, but on the accurate observation and reporting of you, the patient.

There are now in the United Kingdom, many centres which specialise in the diagnosis and treatment of allergic illnesses. In spite of these centres being available, the majority of allergic problems are still probably dealt with by general practitioners. In some ways the general practitioner is in a very good position for getting a good history. The patient probably knows him, and is more relaxed, and is not suffering from the sort of anxiety and tension that comes over so many of us when faced with a hospital visit. The general practitioner can also have access easily to the patient's home if he wants to. He will probably know the patient's immediate family well, and many know, especially in the country areas, about more distant relatives and their health problems. He may also know about the patient's work and the conditions at his work. If your doctor does not send you to a centre for allergies, but at the same time does not get to the bottom of the problem, or supply any real help, you can always ask to be sent for a second opinion.

One of the very real problems of getting a good history is that it is a time-consuming occupation, and if a general practitioner, or a hospital clinic, has short appointment times, there just is not the peace, or the time, for the doctor to get to the bottom of the trouble. This is a problem throughout the Health Service. However, a doctor will do his best, and it helps if the patient can give straightforward answers to questions, and think quickly.

Most allergic reactions, as has been previously explained, are brought about by reaction between an antigen, acting as an allergen, and an antibody. The history and other investigations made, are directed towards unravelling these two parts of the problem. There is no substitute for a thorough history, because other tests may depend on conditions the patient did have, or will have. It must be remembered by both the doctor and patient when getting down to the history, that one patient's trouble may be only partly caused by allergy. He may have another illness as well. It is no good diagnosing and treating the allergy if something more urgent is missed meantime. As 1 in 10 of the entire population of the United Kingdom probably has an allergy, it is very likely that some, especially older patients, have another disease as well. In the infant an allergy of the gut may be diagnosed where in fact the problem is a missing enzyme to digest the milk, or an allergy to wheat cereal may be diagnosed when the infant has a problem called coeliac disease. It is important that both the doctor, and the patient when he is old enough to record his own troubles, should be detailed in giving an account of his symptoms.

A doctor will usually start by asking for the main symptom about which the patient is complaining at the time of the interview. The doctor will then ask about any other symptoms, and particularly whether the symptoms are continuous, or get better or worse. Usually allergic troubles are patchy. There are some times when the patient is all right, or nearly all right, and times when he is very troubled with wheezing or a running nose, or whatever his special problem may be. The patient will then be asked many details about his present symptoms such as what seems to bring them on. He will be asked whether they are worse at any particular time of year, or whether they come on at any time. Sometimes more or less permanent problems may still be worse at certain times. This can happen with an allergic problem of the nose. It may be mostly due to house dust, which is a perennial problem, but can still be made worse in the hay fever season.

If the symptom is seasonal, he will be asked exactly what times of year it comes on. The patient may find this a difficult one to answer if he has only recently had the symptoms, but keeping a diary will probably help for the next year. Different sorts of pollen allergy start at different weeks or months in the year. There is also variation depending on the local climate where you live. In Scotland the hay fever season starts later than in the South of England.

In women the symptoms of an allergic illness may vary according to the time of the menstrual cycle. Some conditions change in severity at puberty, some are worse before the periods, and some change during pregnancy. Some women with asthma are noticeably better during pregnancy. Although these variations occur in a woman's life, there is little known about allergy and hormonal balance.

Symptoms may occur at home, at school or at work. It is important to know when they are worse and when they are better. They may occur more during the week than at the weekend. They may occur only on one day in the week, or only when visiting one particular house. This can happen when there is an allergy to some particular pet which is in the house. The symptoms may be worse out of doors than indoors, or improved while a patient is on holiday. Sometimes the symptoms start after moving to another house, particularly an old one. This can occur where there is an allergy to the house dust mite, or to mould spore. The patient may have improved rapidly when in hospital.

It is important to find out whether symptoms are worse in one particular room in the house such as the attic, the bedroom, or the basement, where dust or mould spores may be implicated. It is also necessary to know whether the symptoms are worse during the day or at night. The blocked nose is commonly more blocked when lying down, and asthmatic attacks are commonest during the night. Therefore symptoms that are worse at night are not necessarily due to an allergen in the bedroom.

It is best if the patient can give all this information spontaneously, but failing this he can be prompted by the doctor. When the answers to all these questions are known, the problem may already be nearing a solution.

The patient is further asked about his past history; whether he was known to have feeding problems or asthma as a baby. All his illnesses and operations in the past need to be recorded. The history of his immediate family may be known to a general practitioner, but will still need to be noted. It is especially important to record whether there is asthma, eczema, or hay fever in the family. It is interesting to find out if there are allergic problems further afield in relatives, than in the immediate family. It is usual to find that there is a positive answer to such enquiries, but with such a high incidence of allergy in the general population this may not mean very much.

If a food allergy is suspected, and the patient is not at all sure which food is accounting for his symptoms, it may be a good idea to note down the foods eaten, and when the symptoms come on. It may become clear that one particular food is the culprit. If, on the other hand, many foods seem to be involved, and there is no one common ingredient such as fish or onion, one must be wary of becoming a food faddist, and avoiding a great number of foods which may not be causing the symptoms, and whose loss may not be good for general health. It is all too easy to become a faddist, and sometimes the doctor can encourage the patient to become one.

The doctor will need to have an account of the patient's previous treatment if he has already had treatment for an allergy. The drugs that helped, and the conditions that helped may make the diagnosis easier. Previous treatment may have made the conditions worse, such as nose drops continued for long periods, or ointments used on eczema or other skin diseases. The bad influence of these treatments may help to muddle up the true diagnosis. The patient may be taking antihistamines at the time he is seen by the doctor, and these will affect skin tests which may be done.

The next step is to do a complete physical examination. This is particularly important in cases of lung disease to rule out other things than allergy. The eyes are examined, and the lining of the nose. In allergic troubles of the nose, the mucosal lining is often a pale colour. The chest will be carefully examined and listened to. The doctor may hear wheezy sounds on deep breathing out. In cases of moderately severe, or severe asthma, the shape of the chest may change, and it may be deeper than normal in an anteroposterior direction. Movements occurring during respiration are less than normal, and it is impossible for the patient to breathe out fully.

The urine is usually examined. This is done as a matter of routine, and largely to exclude diseases other than allergy. In some acute allergic illnesses there may be an increase of protein in the urine. The blood will be examined microscopically. There is often a moderate increase in a particular type of white cell called an eosinophil. The secretion of the eyes and nose may be examined in allergic conditions. These secretions will be clear and colourless. If they are green or yellow the problem is probably an infection and not an allergy, although an infection can be added to an underlying allergy. If the secretions of an allergic condition are stained and examined under a microscope it will be seen that there are a large number of eosinophils.

The history and examination may well have produced a correct diagnosis by the doctor and patient working together. The possible allergens may have been narrowed down to relatively few. The next step may well be skin tests.

In these tests a drop of an extract of the suspected allergen is placed on the skin of the forearm, or on the back, between the shoulder blades. A prick is made through the drop of extract through the superficial layer of the skin with a sterilised needle. In the United Kingdom this is usually the way of doing these tests, but in the United States, scratch tests may be done. There is a possibility of a severe reaction using scratch tests.

Skin tests are usually done to the suspected allergens from the patient's history. Sensitivity to the house dust mite is tested for routinely, and also pollens. Allergy to the house dust mite has been shown to be responsible for many attacks of asthma in the United Kingdom, and also cases of perennial rhinitis, or allergy of the nose. The house dust mite is a small creature, just visible to the naked eye, and related to the spider. It likes warm, damp, dark places, and lives on the scales from human skin. It is a very common inhabitant of bedrooms, and lives on the surface of the mattress and pillows. It is of particular interest, partly because allergy to it causes so much disease, but also because steps taken to keep down the mite population, and desensitize the patient, may have very good results in treatment.

If skin tests are done on skin where there is antibody to the allergen, histamine will be released at the site of the prick, and in 15 to 20 minutes a red weal will appear. Skin tests must be interpreted in the light of the patient's history. He may produce no reaction to allergens which are probably causing his troubles. This can be because the reaction of the skin may be different from the reaction of a sensitized respiratory mucosa. A positive reaction may indicate that a patient has been sensitive to the allergen, but is not necessarily still allergic to it. Multiple allergies shown by skin testing are not as much help in deciding future treatment. Sensitivity which is confined to a few allergens can be of real help to map out a patient's future treatment and management.

In a case of skin disease, known as contact dermatitis, patch testing is done instead of prick testing. Either a piece of the solid, or a piece of gauze soaked in a suspected liquid, is put against the skin and held there by a patch for 24 to 48 hours. If the reaction is red, and possibly blistered, it is positive. If there is discomfort and irritation under the patch at an early stage, then it must be removed and the suspected substance washed off the skin because the patient may be very sensitive to it.

Provocation tests are sometimes used, but should only be done by an expert because of the danger of a severe reaction. They can either be done by putting a spot of the suspected allergen on to the conjunctivae of the eyes, or mucosa of the nose, or in the case of asthma by inhaling the antigen. Measurements of the lung function can be done before and after the test by provocation. It is possible to bring on a very severe attack of asthma by this method, and it is usually possible to make a reliable diagnosis without resorting to such a possibly drastic measure.

In asthma, as part of the investigation of the illness, it is useful to measure the degree to which the lungs function. Because of the changes in asthma that take place in the tubes of the lungs, there is always some impairment to airflow, but it can be useful to know the amount of impairment. This helps to show better than other tests how severe the asthma is, and can also be used as a guide to the effectiveness of a certain line of treatment.

Lung function is usually measured by one of two ways. The total air breathed out, or the forced vital capacity (FVC) can be measured by a simple machine called a Vitalograph. The measurement of the volume of air breathed out in one second is written FEV_1. In the normal person the amount of air breathed out in the first second of expiration is three-quarters or more of the total air breathed out. In asthma this proportion may be considerably reduced. Obstruction to the airways can also be measured by Wright's Peak Flow Meter. A figure for the Peak Flow Rate can be given. This measurement may be made at home, and can be useful for continuous and regular measurement of improvement.

The FEV_1, or the PFR, may be measured before and after the use of a drug to cause broncho-dilatation, or widening of the tubes in the lung. In the case of chronic bronchitis, there will be little or no improvement, but in the case of asthma there may be marked improvement.

Work has been done with these machines on the effect of exercise on asthma. In normal people the result of exercise is to dilate the tubes of the lung, making more air and so more oxygen available to the body. In many asthmatics however, the opposite effect is noticed. Experiments have been done on the effects of running, cycling and swimming in asthmatics. In one survey, 72.5% of people who did running tests, 65% of people who did cycling tests, and 35% of those doing swimming tests, showed a reduced FEV_1 after the exercise. This survey was done in adults. Most asthmatic children show a fall in lung function after exercise. This may continue for many years after the child has no further obvious attacks of asthma. Children may find that different sorts of exercise have a worse effect on them than others. Often cross-country running is worse, and swimming may be the least harmful.

Some doctors believe that a lot of attention should be paid towards emotional factors causing allergy, certainly emotional disturbance plays a part, as will be described in Chapter 16, but probably much of the disturbance is the result of the allergy, and not the cause.

3 General treatment
of allergy

❖❖❖❖

It is not yet possible to stop those with an inherited allergic tendency reacting in one way or another to an allergen, and developing an allergic illness. Therefore, the main lines of treatment are the elimination or avoidance or allergens, or damping down the body's reaction to them. In addition, to these two main lines of help, there is the additional possibility of emotional help from the doctor, or even of psychotherapy. Hypnosis also has been tried, but hypnosis and psychotherapy have little to offer most people who have an allergic illness. It is most important that the patient should have complete confidence in his doctor, understand the treatment he is receiving, and be able to discuss any emotional problems he has. As has been said elsewhere, emotional problems can as often be the result of an allergic disease as the cause of it. The problems that are the result usually are more helped by discussion and the appropriate treatment than the ones that may be considered the causes. General considerations must include diet, rest, exercise, and possibly breathing exercises.

It is necessary before describing the available treatments

for allergies more fully to give a solemn warning. It seldom does good, and more often does harm, to indulge in do-it-yourself cures. A typical example of harm done, is the prolonged use of nose drops for a 'stuffy nose', when in fact the cause is not merely catarrh but an allergic rhinitis. The drops cause a temporary shrinkage of the nasal mucosa, but this is often followed by increased swelling. A further result of prolonged use is the development of polyps in the nose. These may look like bundles of very small grapes and of course, cause further blockage. The presence of polyps can close the entrance to the sinuses or airspaces behind the cheek bones and the forehead. This can lead to infection and more trouble. Another example of damage done by do-it-yourself methods is in the treatment of eczema, or contact dermatitis. Many ointments are powerful sensitizers, and these include ointments containing antihistamines which can be bought without a prescription, and on the face of it look just the thing. These ointments can do a great deal of harm and further complicate the skin disease already present. When in any serious doubt about your health in any way, it is best to consult your doctor.

In the United Kingdom it has only been for the past few years that there has been any widespread interest in the diagnosis and treatment of allergies. Still there are too few centres, and too little time to take the detailed history that was described in the last chapter. Such a history cannot only help to make an accurate diagnosis possible, but can also give a lead in the most effective type of treatment. Failure to make an accurate diagnosis can lead to an unscientific blanket type of treatment just aimed at damping down the body's allergic responses. In some people this may work, but in others it fails, and drugs, often powerful ones, may be taken without due cause.

The first line of treatment should be the elimination, or at least the reduction, of the responsible allergens in the patient's world. Knowing the responsible allergens is obviously of prime importance before effective action can be taken in this connection. A good history and possible confirmation by skin tests may clinch the matter. If it is impossible to eliminate the allergens from the patient's environment, then he should avoid them as far as possible. Pollen and the house dust mite are responsible for many cases of asthma and allergic rhinitis. It is impossible to eliminate these, but they can be reduced to some extent. The patient can take steps to avoid unnecessary exposure to these allergens. Constantly being exposed, far from having a hardening off process, can start to make the allergic reaction more severe. Repeated exposure to large doses of pollen can turn what started as a simple hay fever into pollen induced asthma, which can be a far more severe condition.

Reduction in the exposure to the house dust mite can help to improve many allergic problems, especially asthma. Attention has to be turned first to the bedroom. This is the principle living quarters of the house dust mite, where most of us spend a third or so of our lives. This room must have the closest study and a real attack must be made to eliminate the pest. It lives primarily on the surfaces of the mattress and pillows where it feeds on the scales of human skin which are shed continuously. Having a rubber mattress and pillows will keep down the dust, and make living less comfortable for the house dust mite. If for any reason it is impossible to have a rubber mattress and pillows, others should be covered in polythene. It may be necessary to do this on holiday as a first aid measure, to prevent the possibility of a ruined holiday.

The floor in the bedroom should, if possible, be covered with close fitting lino or other tiles which can be washed and polished regularly. There should be no carpets or mats. Possibly a washable bedside rug may be permitted to make the room less spartan. The curtains and blankets should be washed frequently. There should be no eiderdown or other covering containing feathers or kapok. Everything should be washable at frequent intervals. There should be as little furniture as possible, all that there is should be wiped daily with a damp duster. If possible, all clothes should be kept in cupboards and drawers in another room. The room should be vacuumed daily. It is quite impossible to be rid of all the mites, but reducing the number can cause a remarkable improvement.

These precautions should be taken in other parts of the house where the sufferer goes, but there is a limit to what even the most conscientious housewife can accomplish in the way of keeping her house free of dust. There is some doubt as to whether the more common installation of central heating has had any effect on the mite population. Drying the atmosphere tends to diminish the numbers, but warming it tends to increase them. Paraffin heaters are the worst because they both heat and humidify the atmosphere. Probably conventional types of central heating do little harm as long as windows are opened regularly, and the dust kept down as just described. The exception to opening windows is for the sufferer from hay fever during the hay fever season.

There is always a problem when one of the family develops an allergic disease which is found to be caused by a family pet. It is easy to say that the pet should be removed, but when one seriously considers the role of pets in many homes in the United Kingdom, one realises that the problem is a very difficult one. It may well do more emotional harm than allergic good to dispose of a much loved pet. This question will be discussed more fully in the chapter on Pets and Allergy. This may well be an indication for a course of desensitizing injections.

In allergy to pollen which causes hay fever, it can be extremely difficult to avoid the allergen. Life can be very miserable during the hay fever season for a sufferer who does not have his symptoms controlled, and it does not really help much to live in the centre of a town rather than the country. Pollen can travel many miles in the air, and even a few grains of pollen on the sensitized nasal mucosa can provoke an allergic reaction. June and July are the worst months in England, and the sufferer should preferably sleep with his windows shut. If he must have them open, a screen should be made to fit the window, and covered with a double layer of muslin. Keeping the muslin damp probably makes it more effective as a screen against pollen. It is best to avoid vases of flowers or grasses in the house.

The hay fever victim must keep away from all grassy

places during the pollen season, including school playing fields, golf courses, and all open grassy places. Outings to the country and picnics are best avoided. If it is necessary to drive the car through the country, it is best to keep the windows shut. Holidays are best avoided in June and July, because they may be spoilt by symptoms getting worse. Ideally, a long sea cruise should be taken during the bad weeks, but not many of us can afford that luxury. Seaside holidays are better than country holidays, and holidays at high altitudes seem to be better than at lower altitudes.

Sometimes, asthma or allergic rhinitis may be due to mould spores. These can grow on the leaves of plants, especially in a hot house where there is a warm, damp atmosphere. If a sensitivity to mould spores is suspected or confirmed on skin testing, the house, and especially a basement or cellar, should be searched for damp places which can be treated. This type of allergy will not be seasonal.

Allergy to some substances such as mouldy hay, may be met in the course of work. Sometimes these allergies are very difficult to treat and eventually it may be necessary for a doctor to advise his patient to change his occupation. Obviously, this advice would not be given until all other avenues had been explored and failed to supply an answer. In middle age especially, advice to change an occupation would not be given without very good reason. In food allergies, where the affecting food is known for certain, it should be avoided. It may be found that after a time of complete avoidance it can be tolerated again in small quantities. This can occur in an infant allergic to cow's milk. In an infant who is allergic to cow's milk, it may be necessary to use a milk substitute, and it is important to remember to use a substitute for mixing cereals. Sometimes boiling cow's milk gently for 10 minutes has a sufficient effect on the proteins to avoid an allergic reaction.

It is not usually possible to control an allergic reaction completely by avoiding or reducing the amount of allergen with which the patient comes in contact. It is usually also necessary to damp down the body's way of acting in an allergic fashion. One of the common, and often effective ways of doing this, is by taking antihistamines. These tablets, or medicines, counteract the action of histamine which is released in the allergic reaction. There are many antihistamine preparations on the market and the chief differences in them is the length of their action, and the number of side effects they produce in the individual patient. All antihistamines have some sedative action, but the effect on any particular person can only be found by trying the drug. The patient should be warned not to drive a vehicle or operate any machinery after he has taken such a drug, until he is assured of its effects on him. In children, when often a sedative effect might be welcomed in an allergic condition, there is least reaction in this direction.

Antihistamines are most useful in hay fever and allergic rhinitis. They are also sometimes helpful in slow release preparations, and one of these taken at night may be effective throughout the day as well, and not cause undue drowsiness at a time when it is not required. Antihistamines do not usually have any beneficial effect in asthma, even when it is known to be allergic asthma.

Desensitizing injections have been in use for many years. They were started by a Doctor Noon in 1911. At first a solution of allergen in water was used, and at least 20 injections were necessary, but now there are new injections available, and not so many need be given. The present theory of action of desensitizing injections is that they make the patient's body produce what can be called a 'blocking antibody'. These antibodies are another of the immunoglobulins. They are in the blood and are mobile. When a potential allergen comes into contact with the body, these blocking antibodies meet it and defuse it before it can meet an allergic antibody. This prevents an allergic reaction occurring. More scientifically it is known that there is an increase of one immunoglobulin IgG and the decrease in IgE during the process of densensitization.

The best results of desensitization are obtained when one or two antigens are found to be the culprits. Then a solution can be given against these. The worst results are obtained when there are apparently multiple allergens and a desensitizing cocktail is given. This has to be made specially, it is very expensive, it means 20 injections, and it usually is disappointing in results.

Desensitizing injections are indicated in several situations. The first is hay fever or other pollen allergy which has not responded to several measures including antihistamines. The injections used against pollens are alum precipitated ones and a course of about eight have to be given at weekly intervals. An emulsion can be used and only three or four injections given at monthly intervals. The trouble with the latter is the likelihood of a sterile abscess forming at the site of the injection. Anybody with hay fever which has not responded to antihistamines should see his doctor in the autumn. This leaves enough time for investigation of the allergy to be done and the course of injections to be finished before the start of the hay fever season. In the United Kingdom it is not usual to give desensitizing injections during the hay fever season.

If hay fever is allowed to continue there is always the chance of pollen asthma developing. There is about an 80% success in desensitization against grass pollen. Unfortunately, even if successful the injections have to be continued for several years. After that there may be a permanent improvement. Allergy to common mould spores may also be helped by a course of injections. In recent years it has been found that desensitization to the house dust mite can be very effective in asthma and allergic rhinitis. It has been estimated that up to three-quarters of Britain's asthmatics could be helped by this type of desensitization. Formerly it was difficult to produce an extract for injection because the house dust mite is a very choosy feeder, difficult to breed away from its natural environment. However, the problem has now been overcome. The last good reason for desensitization is allergy to bee or wasp stings, where there has been a severe general reaction. This is one of the hazards of allergy that cannot be catered for by drugs in a preventive way.

The main reason for not desensitizing somebody is that he has had a severe reaction during a previous course of injections. If somebody has a mild reaction, possibly with sneezing or an itching skin, the dose is not increased at the next injection, and the patient may be advised to take an antihistamine tablet before the injection. Desensitization is not usually done in children under five. Between the ages of 5–12, it is only done after discussion with the child.

There are various drugs that are used in asthma which have the effect of dilating the passages in the lungs. These are collectively called bronchodilators. They may be sucked in the mouth, swallowed, inhaled as an aerosol, or injected. It is possible, but not usual now, to give some as suppositories in the back passage. Some asthma, which is not severe, responds to ephedrine, or more recently salbutamol, taken by mouth. Isoprenaline can be dissolved under the tongue. It can be effective, but can cause palpitations and also may cause soreness of the mouth.

Isoprenaline can also be used as an aerosol. This was used frequently but during the 1960's there was a rise in the number of deaths caused by asthma and this was connected with the increasing use of bronchodilator aerosols. The reason behind this may have been some ill effect on the heart, or it may have been the patients and doctors who were relying on these aerosols when really the asthma was too severe to respond, and other more drastic treatment was indicated. If a patient is prescribed such an aerosol, he must be told the maximum number of doses he can have, and that this must not be exceeded. If his asthma does not respond to the usual dose, then it must not be increased, but he must get medical help. Used properly, these aerosols are of great help to many people, and if not used in excessive dosage, are not dangerous.

Adrenalin can be given by injection in severe cases of asthma, or in anaphylactic shock. Antihistamines can also be given by injection in severe urticaria, or nettle-rash, of the skin, anaphylaxis or serum sickness.

A new drug has become available for the prevention of allergy in the past five years. It was first discovered in 1967 that disodium cromoglycate interfered with the allergic reaction. The first three letters of interfered—INT, and the first two letters of allergic—AL, gave it the trade name

Intal. It is used in the prevention and not directly in the treatment of allergic reaction. Therefore, it has to be used regularly for the necessary length of time to show its real effect. Its way of acting is not fully understood, but it is believed to act on the membranes covering the mask cells, making them more stable and less likely to break up and release histamine on contact with an allergen. It is of more use in an allergic asthma than in other kinds of asthma. Even so, not all people with allergic asthma are helped, and the reasons for this are not known. It is usual to give Intal a month's trial in any individual, and if there is no improvement in that time, to discontinue it.

The drug is given in the form of a capsule which is inhaled as powder through a gadget called a spinhaler. When the drug was first used it was combined with Isoprenaline and was called Intal Co. Now, it is more usual to use Intal alone. If the drug is effective, it is usual to reduce the dose to the minimum which will control the symptoms. It is often effective in preventing exercise-induced asthma, particularly in children. To decide whether improvement has taken place, it is useful if the patient or the parent, if the patient is a child, keeps a diary noting the number and the severity of the attacks, and also the number of other drugs necessary to control the symptoms. Disodium cromoglycate can be used in the treatment of allergic rhinitis in the form of Rynacrom. It is more effective in hay fever than in perennial allergic rhinitis.

In some children with severe asthma who are taking steroids regularly, the introduction of Intal meant between a quarter and half the children could be taken off steroids.

Perhaps the most important drugs in the treatment of severe allergy are the steroids. These drugs can be used as creams, ointments, or sprays for the skin, or can be taken as tablets by mouth, can be inhaled, used as nose drops, or injected. They are a powerful weapon in the hand of the doctor to be used when and if really necessary. They can be life saving if injected into a vein in very severe asthma. However, they are never used lightly, because once started by mouth or injection, it may be difficult to get a patient off them, and they may have serious side-effects. They are not used in patients who have a gastric or duodenal ulcer, diabetes, or tuberculosis. The patient should be warned that if, while on them, he gets any infection he should seek medical advice. Steroids suppress, not only the making of allergic antibodies, but also the making of immune antibodies, and therefore, if the patient gets any infection he will probably need to take an antibiotic.

Steroids can have serious side effects. Given regularly to children, even in small doses, they slow up growth in about one-third of children. In adults they can cause an increase in weight, and a change in the shape of the face, sometimes called a 'moon face'.

Recently, an aerosol steroid has been introduced called beclomethazone dipropionate which is proving to be very effective in some allergic conditions. Patients must be properly instructed in its use. It is very important that the patient is told at the beginning of treatment exactly how to use it. He must breathe out fully, and then release the capsule at the beginning of a sudden deep inspiration. In this way the small particles of powder are drawn down as far as possible into the lungs. It seems to have the advantages of steroids without the unwanted side effects. It is very active on the surfaces of the body that show allergic reactions, but does not seem to have any other effects on the body. Some patients started on this can be weaned off steroids by mouth, but they should always have steroids available in case of a severe attack.

Beclomethasone dipropionate is most effective in the treatment of allergic asthma. Tests for lung function sometimes show an improvement following its use. It is, however, sometimes useful in patients with asthma who are not allergic. It is usual to give it a month's trial with 4 capsules daily, and if there is no improvement in a month it is stopped. As for the trial of Intal it is very helpful if the patient keeps a diary. Recently, beclomethazone dipropionate nasal spray has been introduced for the treatment of hay fever and allergic rhinitis.

In addition to the use of drugs and desensitization there

are other more general treatments for allergic conditions. Some people believe that breathing exercises can be very helpful in the treatment of asthma. Certainly they do seem to work for some patients and there is no harm in giving them a try. These exercises are discussed in more detail in Chapter 4 on Asthma. Attention should always be paid to general health. This includes taking a good mixed diet without too much flour and sugar, having adequate rest and as much fresh air and exercise as possible.

There is a lot of doubt about the effectiveness of psychotherapy and hypnosis in the treatment of allergic conditions. It is certain that there is an element which is not physical about some allergies. It is known for a person to get hay fever when just shown a picture of grass. There is always a great need for a sufferer to have confidence in his doctor and to get sufficient support through the rough patches. This question will be discussed more fully in the chapter on Allergy and the Mind.

4 Asthma

❖❖❖❖

There is still no generally accepted definition of asthma, although the disease has been recognised and described since the earliest days of medicine. Probably the best definition includes the facts that asthma is a disease which has attacks of breathlessness. This is due to narrowing and blocking of the lung airways which is usually and completely reversible either by itself, or because of treatment. Attacks of breathlessness occur in many other diseases, but not from the same causes. Most attacks of asthma would clear up by themselves but the clearing-up can be speeded by the right treatment.

There are various estimates of the number of asthmatics in the United Kingdom. A guarded estimate is that 2% of the total population have asthma. It is more probable that nearly 5% have asthma. This makes it one of the most common potentially crippling diseases. There are probably about 2 million asthmatics in the United Kingdom. Asthma can start at any age from a few months old up to over 60 years of age. About one third of cases start during the first 10 years of life, and it is relatively rare to start over the age of

60. The diagnosis is always more difficult to make in the older aged people because of the likelihood of other troubles such as high blood pressure and bronchitis which could be responsible for similar symptoms. Asthma can be very difficult to distinguish from bronchitis. In babies the diagnosis can be muddled with wheezy bronchitis, but as will be described more fully in the Chapter 5 on Asthma in Children, this is very likely to be part of the same illness, especially in view of the similar family history of allergy. In older people, the diagnosis of asthma is sometimes made when wheezing starts. This should not be done because the treatment is different and the blockage of the lung tubes will often be relieved quite effectively in asthma, but not in long-standing bronchitis.

The person with bronchitis is very often a smoker, and the asthmatic may often not smoke at all. Chronic bronchitis in a non-smoker can happen but it is rare. Those with asthma, even if late in starting, may have a family history of allergy or a personal history of allergy such as hay fever occurring earlier in their own lives. Both in bronchitis and in asthmatics the wheezing may only start after an infection with the upper respiratory tract such as a cold, or an attack of sinusitis. In asthma the blockage of the airways is largely reversible and a trial may be made with drugs such as steroids. There is no similar response in bronchitis. Tests on the function in the lungs show in asthma that the function is improved by drugs and usually worsened by exercise. Again this may not be so in people suffering from bronchitis.

Asthma usually comes on suddenly and normally there is no fever and the sputum is clear mucous sputum. Bronchitis usually comes on gradually, there is normally a fever, and when the bronchitis is fully developed the sputum is thick and yellow. Occasionally the first attack of asthma can start as a complication of bronchitis, and the diagnosis is then very difficult to make, indeed it is often not possible at this first attack, but the subsequent events will show that asthma has started.

Blood and sputum tests can help to distinguish between asthma and bronchitis. In asthma, both in the blood and the sputum there are an increased number of a type of white blood cell called eosinophils. This increase is usual in various types of allergy, including hay fever and allergic rhinitis. Both asthma and bronchitis, unless adequately and effectively treated in the early stages, can cause permanent damage to the lungs. This means that the amount of air, and in particular oxygen which the patient can breathe in may be severely reduced and there may be constant breathlessness. The causes of asthma can be many, but are usually grouped under the three headings of allergic, infective and psychological. Here we are mainly concerned with the allergic causes. Asthma is sometimes labelled psychological in origin, but it is very doubtful if psychological or emotional upsets are ever the only cause of asthma. It can occur, however, that an acute domestic or business worry can trigger off an attack in somebody already prone to asthma. It is quoted that somebody who is allergic to dogs can get an attack of asthma on being shown a picture of a dog. Psychotherapy and hypnosis have been tried in treating asthma by those who believe in psychological causes, but there has been little concrete proof of any success.

It is possible that endocrine causes have some part in starting asthma attacks. In young women they may occur in the premenstrual phase of the menstrual cycle, and in older women there may be severe attacks of asthma during the menopause. Sometimes the menopausal asthma is believed to be associated with a menopausal depression, and treatment of the depression can help the asthma. Even so, the asthma is basically due to the patient's make-up and not due to psychological causes. The young woman with asthma may improve dramatically during pregnancy, and this is possibly due to hormonal change. After the delivery of the baby the asthma again may get a lot worse.

Asthma has more emotional results than emotional causes. It may cause a great deal of frustration in limiting a person's activities, especially if he is ambitious. Both his business and his social activities may have to be curbed, and the sufferer may have to put up with bouts of incapacitating illness. The long-term outlook for the severe adult asthmatic is, it must be said, beset with difficulties. Frequent attacks of asthma cause much disturbance to sleep, and possibly chronic tiredness.

Infection may cause attacks of asthma, and attacks may always occur after a cold. It is usual in such people that there is some family history of allergy, and in the patients themselves there is some allergic tendency. It is impossible, especially in the climate of the United Kingdom to avoid infection of the upper respiratory tract. At this time there is no really effective way of preventing colds, and the subsequent attacks of asthma just have to be dealt with as they occur. Routine antibiotics given with colds have not been shown to be effective in preventing an attack of asthma.

Allergic causes are probably the most common causes of asthma. 50% of asthmatics have a family history of allergy. The chances of asthma occurring in the first degree relatives of an asthmatic is 50% before the age of 65 years. In asthmatics there is an increased changeability in size of the air tubes in the lungs which is known as bronchial hyperactivity. There is also the reaction that has been described previously. Sensitized cells in the lining of the respiratory tubes are affected by the presence of an allergen. The allergen may be one of many things, but it is often some sort of protein. It may vary from pollen to the house dust mite. When the allergen lands on the sensitized cells histamine is set free and acts in three ways. First histamine causes swelling of the lining of the tubes, secondly it causes contraction of the muscle surrounding the tubes, and thirdly it causes a thick secretion from the mucous glands in the lining of the tubes of the lung. All these three act to narrow the bronchial tubes in the lung, and so make it more difficult to give the air a free passage through the lung.

An attack of asthma usually comes on suddenly. Normally breathing in is an active process when the muscles between the ribs contract and the diaphragm moves downwards. Breathing out is passive, and the muscles and diaphragm relax. In asthma, breathing out is the problem because of the blocked tubes. It needs a positive effort on the part of the patient to get air out of the lung, and the passage of the air may be accompanied by a wheezing sound which can be heard easily from some distance. The muscles in the neck which are called the accessory muscles of respiration will probably contract in an effort to force air out of the lungs. The patient is usually more comfortable sitting up and this may make breathing out easier. At the beginning of the attack there may be coughing with no sputum, but towards the end of the attack mucoid sputum may usually be coughed up. Sometimes this sputum comes up in plugs the shape of the bronchial tubes it has been blocking.

With efficient treatment an attack of asthma can be shortened, but usually it will pass whether it is treated or not. Attacks occur most commonly at night. Sometimes, however, the attack does not clear up with the usual treatment, or by itself. The effort of forcing the air out of the lungs can cause additional narrowing of the tubes and a vicious circle is set up. The patient seems to be making less respiratory effort and his breathing may become very shallow; he may have been wheezing for some hours and have been without food or drink, he becomes exhausted, and this is called status asthmaticus and needs immediate medical help and admission to hospital. When the diagnosis of asthma is made your doctor will usually decide at what point he should be called in if an attack does not respond to treatment.

Asthma can be diagnosed by your doctor in various ways. He will first take a good history of your own complaints, including particularly the things that you have noticed bring on attacks. This may include sleeping in a different bed, working in the greenhouse, or it may only occur while you are at work. The doctor will make a thorough note about your past history, and particularly of any allergy, and of your family history. He may make further investigations himself, or he may refer you to a specialist. He will probably do this if attacks are severe and interfere with your life and work.

The specialist will also take a history which may give him some clue about the cause of the asthma, for example the introduction of a dog to the household. He will have a chest X-ray done and an examination of blood and sputum. He will probably arrange for prick tests to be done for known or probable allergens. These are done on the back, between the shoulder blades, or on the forearm, and about 12 are done at a time. A drop of the extract of the allergen is put on the skin, and a prick made in the middle of it. If any allergen is causing the asthma it will show a reaction in about 20 minutes. The allergens most commonly used are pollens, house dust mite, animal dander and in some cases food if this seems applicable. Allergies to milk, fish or egg may occur, and cause asthma, sometimes accompanied by skin reactions. It is important to be aware of putting too much emphasis on food allergens if there are a great number of them because it can very easily lead to food faddism.

The specialist will probably do tests for the function of the lungs. This can be done on several devices, but the two most usual measurements are known as the Peak Expiratory Flow Rate which is measured with Wright's Peak Flow Meter, and the Forced Expiratory Volume which is measured during one second and is known as the FEV_1. The latter is particularly useful in measuring accurately the response to any treatment and the improvement or worsening in a patient's asthma. The FEV_1 can be measured before and after the inhalation of a drug to dilate the bronchial passages, and if there is no improvement the drug is likely to be ineffective. Sometimes asthma is brought on by exercise and this can be shown scientifically by measuring the FEV_1 before and after exercise.

There are many drugs used in the treatment of asthma. In mild asthma tablets of ephedrine, or salbutamol, may be adequate. These are simple bronchodilators and can be taken by mouth. Bronchodilators may also be used in aerosol form. This used to be a very popular way of treating asthma, but if used in too large a dose damage can be done to the heart. These aerosols are still used, but it is very important that the exact dose should be laid down by the doctor and obeyed by the patient. If during an acute attack of asthma there is no response to the aerosol the maximum dose should never be exceeded.

In the past few years a new approach has been made in the

drug treatment of asthma. This drug is disodium cromoglycate, marketed as Intal, which is essentially a preventive and the patient must be told to use it regularly whether he is wheezing or not. It is thought to act by making the sensitive cells in the bronchial mucosa less sensitive and not so likely to break down and release histamine when they come into contact with an allergen. It is usually given in a spinhaler and at first used four times daily. If it is effective the dose may be gradually reduced. If there is no improvement after using it for a month it is unlikely to be effective.

If all else fails steroids may be given. In children a short course may be given and then gradually stopped. Adults, once started on steroids, are not very likely to get off them. They may be given by mouth or injection, or more recently by inhalation as a snuff. Steroids given by mouth and injection can have undesirable side effects such as weight gain and rise in blood pressure. Steroids given as an inhalation are called beclomethasone dipropionate. This looks as though it is going to be very useful. The only side effects seem to be thrush in the mouth and throat. The patient must be shown carefully how to use it so that the maximum amount of steroid powder gets to the smaller lung passages.

When a diagnosis of asthma is made the patient should have plenty of opportunity of discussing all his problems with an understanding doctor. Any emotional problems should be sympathetically discussed, and if possible sorted out. If asthma occurs for the first time later in life, the first attack may be very distressing and the patient and his family gets in a state of panic. If they have a chance of discussing the treatment and general management of asthma they may feel less worried and the calmer situation will probably benefit the patient.

If the allergen is known it may be possible to avoid it, for example if it is an animal. If this is not possible, desensitization may be done. In general desensitization is disappointing, apart from desensitization to the house dust mite.

It is important that as far as possible the asthmatic should live in a dust free atmosphere. He should have a dunlopillow mattress and pillows. The mattress should be covered with polythene and vacuumed regularly. All bedding, including blankets and the curtains in the room should be laundered regularly. Carpets should be avoided and furniture kept to a minimum. All surfaces should be wiped daily with a damp duster. The asthmatic usually benefits from living in an even temperature, going from a warm living room to a cold bedroom can trigger off an attack. The bedroom should be warmed before going to bed. On the other hand, overheating can have a bad effect. Putting central heating into a house which dries the air can make asthma worse.

Asthma can be caused by moulds which may occur in a greenhouse or at work. Farmers are particularly likely to get a type of asthma from the mould which grows in damp hay, but this will be described more fully in the chapter on occupational allergies. If an allergen at work is causing asthma it may be necessary to change your job, but this is only done as a last resort. If a known food is causing an allergy it should be avoided. In general, during an asthmatic attack small amounts of food and drink should be given. All aerated drinks should be avoided. No asthmatic should smoke, and should whenever possible avoid a smoky atmosphere.

Breathing exercises may help particularly if a patient can be taught to breathe more with his diaphragm and less with the other part of his chest. This is best learnt lying flat on his back with a piece of paper on his tummy and then seeing how far up and down he can move the piece of paper.

The sufferer from asthma should know about status asthmaticus, and should be told clearly by his doctor at what point he should call for medical help if the attack of asthma does not respond to the usual treatment. Anybody with status asthmaticus must be admitted to hospital for intensive treatment following first aid by his doctor at home.

Asthma gives a feeling of tightness and discomfort in the chest, but it does not cause pain. If there is pain, it means that there is probably some complication, and your doctor should be told about it at once.

Asthma, which starts in adult life, can certainly be helped a lot with medical advice, but the tendency to asthma is likely to remain and the sufferer will have to learn to live with it.

5 Your child
and asthma

❖❖❖❖❖

Children may develop most of the types of allergy that an adult may develop. Because they are young, and because of your close relationship with them, some of the problems posed are a bit different. The ways in which allergies are caused have already been described, and these are essentially the same in a child. There are, however, probably more emotional problems with a child's allergy. For a mother it is much more anxiety making for her child to have asthma than to have asthma herself. It is very easy for a doctor to say that a mother becomes overprotective and overanxious, but it is difficult to see how any conscientious parent could avoid doing just this.

About one-third of all long-standing illness in children is due to allergy of one sort or another. The most common reason for long absence from school is asthma. Allergies of all sorts are illnesses that are difficult to cure. They may be prevented and relieved, but in the long term they have to be lived with. It is very difficult to accept that a child with so many years ahead of him may have a handicapping illness to live with. Many allergies do improve with time, but nevertheless it may be many years before the child is free, and the tendency remains.

It is very important that a child should get the best possible investigation and treatment so that he may have a good chance of recovering before he leaves school, otherwise a child with asthma enters adult life as a handicapped person if the asthma is at all severe. Sometimes vaccines are used, but usually unscientifically and with few beneficial results. This is partly because of the shortage of doctors with a special knowledge of allergy in the United Kingdom. It is reckoned that with proper investigation and treatment more than 70% of children with asthma could be cleared of the problem by the time they leave school.

Asthma is the most frequent and can be the most handicapping of the allergies in childhood. It has been estimated that there are about 150,000 children in the United Kingdom who will have asthma at some time during their childhood. As many as 1 in 10 have a wheezy attack at some time before the age of 10 years, but many of them grow out of it after this age. A child who has had frequent attacks of wheezing before the age of three years, particularly if these attacks are not all associated with a cold, is more likely to have to learn to live with asthma for a longer time. He is certainly more likely to have asthma after the age of 10 years. It has been estimated that 4% of all children will remain asthmatics, so that it is a very common cause of childish ill-health. For some unknown reason boys are twice as likely as girls to be asthmatics.

It is not exactly known in what way heredity and asthma work together; as 10% of the population have an allergy of some sort or another it can be seen that the incidence in one family might be coincidental. Studies of identical twins have shown that they are four times as likely to both have asthma as non-identical twins, so there is some evidence that it is inherited. Certainly doctors find that hay fever, eczema and asthma all go together in families. A baby may develop eczema and later this may improve, and he may start having asthma. There does seem to be what may be described as allergic stock but it may take trigger factors, such as infection or an emotional shock to start off an allergic illness.

It is possibly doubtful whether all small children of say under three years of age who wheeze after a cold should be called asthmatics. It is probable that it is all the same illness, but two out of three of these children will be clear of symptoms by the age of seven years. If the parents do not have an allergy, and if the child has not had eczema, it is probable that he can be called just a wheezy baby, and he will grow out of it. It can be very upsetting for a mother if a doctor makes a diagnosis of asthma at the first wheezy illness; to her it conjures up a picture of gloom, and a long life of invalidism. She feels anxious and worried, and inevitably some of the worry rubs off on the child.

Asthma that starts before the age of three years is more likely to continue, especially if the attacks get more frequent and are not related to colds. Probably half of these children will be clear by the age of 10 years, but the other half will continue to have attacks into adult life, and possibly always have them. Asthma is more likely to continue if there is a high frequency of attacks during the first year after the onset. There is also more likelihood of the asthma continuing if there is permanent impairment of lung function as shown by tests. It is also more likely to continue if chest deformity develops. The deformity most likely to develop is an increase of the chest from fore to aft, resulting in what has been described as a barrel shaped chest. Mild asthma often starts later in childhood. The attacks occur at infrequent intervals, and the child is completely free from wheezing between attacks. Up to 40% of small children with eczema will have an attack of asthma before the age of 6 years.

Asthma has three likely causes in childhood, and these are infective, allergic, and emotional. Infective causes usually show themselves after a cold. Children do have colds very frequently, especially during their first years at school, so that it can be seen that these attacks of wheezing may be very frequent. It is not advisable to remove tonsils and adenoids from an asthmatic child and there is no evidence that their removal improves the asthma. Some children are given routine antibiotics at the beginning of colds, but most authorities agree now that this does not help.

There may be an allergic cause for asthma, although it can be very difficult to sort out. The best way of finding an allergic cause is by your doctor taking a very careful history, and you being a very accurate observer. It could be that your child only gets attacks of asthma on Sunday when he goes to see granny who has a dog, and that would show that he is sensitive to the dander of the dog's fur. In this case it would not be wise to stop him seeing granny or make her get rid of the dog, but he could have a dose of medicine before the visit.

Other observations that you make about the time of the year when the attacks occur, or a change of house, may help your doctor. It has been shown recently that some asthma is due to the house dust mite dermatophagoides pteronyssius. This mite is more often found in old houses; it is a type of arachnid, a relation of the spider, and is just visible to the naked eye. It feeds on the scales from the human skin and likes a warm, moist atmosphere which is often found on the surfaces of mattresses. If the surface of the mattress is vacuum cleaned and a plastic sheet is spread over it, it keeps the mite down.

Skin tests to different substances causing allergies are not very satisfactory. The tests are done on the skin and there is a difference between the reaction of the skin to these dusts and the reaction of the lungs when the substances are breathed in. Sometimes the child is found to be very sensitive to one particular thing such as feathers, and a change to a Dunlopillo mattress and pillows may make a big improvement, but other times a child is found to be allergic to a family pet. This always poses a great problem and the emotional damage done by getting rid of the pet will far outweigh any possible advantage. The best advice is usually not to replace the pet when he dies. The possible exception to skin sensitivity, and the possibility of desensitization is allergy to the house dust mite. In one trial 77% of 150 children with a history of all-the-year-round asthma gave a positive result to skin tests with an extract of house dust mite. This sort of asthma is often relieved by admission to hospital. Sometimes it can be mistakenly attributed to the child getting away from home influences and parental anxieties, but it is just as likely that it is due to getting away from the home house dust mite.

Desensitizing is not usually much help. It means a very prolonged course of injections which are usually upsetting to a child and there may not be much improvement. A new vaccine has been produced against the house dust mite which may be of value, but it is not yet known just how effective it will be.

There are usually emotional factors with asthma, but emotional problems are very seldom the only cause. It is very easy for a mother or for both parents to be labelled as over-protective and overanxious, but until one has watched a small child wheezing his way through an attack of asthma, it is not possible to understand just how natural and inevitable these reactions are. Sometimes an upset family does have an effect on the child, and the solution of a marital problem, even if it means divorce, can have a very beneficial effect on the child and his asthma. If you as a mother know that you have emotional problems of your own, obviously in the interests of your child you must discuss these with somebody, preferably your doctor, and get help in sorting them out.

Referral to a psychiatrist before the child has been properly investigated for the causes of his asthma, can cause the whole situation to get worse. The referral can add to the parents' guilt that their child is ill and it increases the suggestion that they are in some way responsible. The mother may be labelled as rejecting or overprotective and it may be suggested that her attitude is the cause of the child's illness. It is far more likely that any emotional problems she may show are the result and not the cause of her child's asthma.

You can get very tired from coping with frequent attacks of asthma at night. Tiredness does not help. Your doctor should be able to help you with these problems. You should be able to tell him about your worries and fears. He should be able to find the time to listen to your problems and explain all the facts of asthma to you, and how you can best help your child. It is often a help to see a child specialist who may be able to suggest improved management of your child. If your doctor does not suggest such a visit then it is quite in order for you to ask for a second opinion. In the last resort, if you do not get the help and support you need from your doctor you may have to find a more understanding doctor.

Parents need to gain self-confidence in coping with a child with asthma. If the treatment is right and you understand that the illness can only be helped and not cured you will be able by a positive outlook to give your child more self-confidence.

There are many treatments available for asthma. You should realise, however, that treatment of asthma is aimed at preventing attacks and making them less severe. It will not actually cure the asthma, although sometimes it seems able to do that. Treatment should be managed so that it interferes as little as possible with your child's growth and development. It should be geared so that he can lead as normal and as independent a life as possible. Once you have found a doctor you can trust you must help him all you can to help your child to achieve an independent existence. When he is old enough he will be able to manage his own treatment to a large extent.

There are many drugs used in the milder attacks of asthma, including ephedrine and salbutamol (Ventolin). Many doctors do not recommend the use of aminophyline rectal suppositories, although some use them for attacks at night. Sprays containing dilators of the small lung tubes can sometimes be helpful, but are not used as frequently now as 15 years ago. If they are used it is very important that the doctor lays down the maximum dosage to be used, and also explains the limitations of the spray to help a very severe attack of asthma.

The latest drug used in the prevention of an attack of asthma is disodium cromoglycate (Intal). This is not used in the treatment of an attack, but is for use all the time for prevention. It is an extremely useful drug for many children, but in some it has no effect.

In serious chronic asthma, or in very acute attacks, steroids may be used. They are extremely effective in cutting short severe attacks, or in bringing to an end a long lasting wheezy spell. There is little harm in using them for short spells. There are, however, very real dangers in using them for long periods. The child can become dependent on them and if used for a very long time in largish dosage they can retard a child's physical growth.

If a child has a very severe attack of asthma he may be admitted to hospital where he can be given intensive treatment, including oxygen therapy. You should always have an arrangement with your doctor at what stage you call him in if the attack does not respond to the usual treatment.

Breathing and relaxation exercises are advised by some doctors and do seem to help some children. It is important that you should learn the exercises with your child and practise them with him at frequent intervals.

Your child should go to school as much as possible. It is very easy to keep him away from school because he is wheezing and you feel it may get worse. More often the wheeze will get better once he gets to school, and he should only be kept away if he is really ill. It is particularly important that an asthmatic child's school attendance should be as good as possible. His future will be very dependent on adequate academic success. Often he will not be fit for unskilled work. If he starts missing school he gets behind in work, then he starts worrying about going to school because he is behind, and the worry makes him worse. It has been shown that asthmatic children tend to be of above average intelligence which is a further reason why they should get all the education possible. Many asthmatic children manage to get over their earlier handicap and possibly poor school attendance and get to university. Because they are often made worse by an active hobby they tend to become interested in reading, model making and sometimes music, and these interests should be encouraged.

You should have contact with your child's teachers and the School Medical Officer. They should know what drugs he is having, and know how much he may have in a certain time. The child should have as full a life as possible at school. He is the best judge of what he is capable. Sometimes one particular activity such as cross-country running can bring on an attack of asthma and this should be avoided. He can usually do all indoor physical activity and swimming, and he should be encouraged to do this. One survey on asthma, brought on by exercise, showed that asthma occurred in 72.5% of those surveyed after running tests, 65% after cycling tests and only 35% after swimming tests. Swimming should obviously be recommended as exercise for asthmatic children rather than running sports or cycling.

Sometimes a residential school is advised. The improvement in a child can be dramatic, but he often gets worse when he returns home. Naturally, this makes the parents feel very inadequate and sometimes guilty. If a child does go away it is very important that the parents should not be left to brood about the problem on their own but should be given real help and advice while he is away and enough support when he returns home.

A child from a family which has strong allergic tendencies should keep in as dust free an atmosphere as possible. This needs to be done with as little fussing as is possible. Asthma in a child can be a very depressing and anxiety making illness. It is important that you should try to be confident and optimistic, having done all that is prescribed by your doctor, hope can be a great help. Time is on your side and many children will grow out of their asthma.

Strictly speaking, hay fever is seasonal irritation of the lining of the nose and eyes caused by grass pollen. In actual fact the term hay fever is used to cover a much greater variety of troubles than the strict definition implies. It is always seasonal, but as well as grass pollen it includes pollen from other weeds, and spores from some moulds. In the United States it also includes the pollen from rag weed which is a serious offender and which comes later in the year than the pollen from grasses. Hay fever is not really a very good description of this illness because it is not caused just by hay and does not cause a fever.

In the United States it has been reckoned that between 5 and 10% of the population have hay fever. The number of people with hay fever has not been estimated in the United Kingdom, but it is possibly not such a large number because rag weed does not grow in the United Kingdom.

Hay fever may be accompanied by allergy of the nose to other things which continues throughout the year and this may make diagnosis difficult. In some people there may be no symptoms from the nose but only a reaction in the eyes.

When children have this they tend to rub their itchy eyes causing swelling and infection, and a diagnosis of 'pink eye' can be mistakenly made. It may be only when it is realised that the symptoms come at the same time each year that the correct diagnosis is made.

Hay fever, unlike many other types of allergic illness, is almost a pure allergy. Infective and psychological causes do not play much part, although occasionally it is found that emotional upsets can affect the lining of the nose. Hay fever is caused by the lighter pollens and mould spores which are easily airborne. These include grasses, nettles, some trees such as plane and silver birch, willow and beech can cause it. In the United Kingdom 90% of the trouble is caused by grass pollens. This starts in late May and goes on until the middle of July. The worst weeks are usually the last week of June and the first week of July. In the North of England and Scotland, these times may be up to a fortnight later. It can be seen that these times coincide with many public examinations. It is hardly possible for a child to do his best in an examination while suffering from hay fever. It has been pointed out to the Examination Boards, but so far no change has been made.

In the United Kingdom 72% of patients with hay fever start between the ages of 5 and 20, so it is very much a problem of the older child and young adult. The first time that somebody goes to the doctor with it, the trouble may be diagnosed as a common cold. However, the following year it may start at almost exactly the same day and a proper diagnosis is made. 60% of people with hay fever have a history of other allergic problems, most commonly asthma and eczema. These may be in the past or they may still have them. There is a family history of allergies in more than half of those people with hay fever. Hay fever tends to improve over the years, and often it disappears after about 40 years of age, but it is poor comfort to a boy of 15 years to be told to be patient for 25 years or more and the problem will clear up. Something much more active must be done meantime.

Allergy to mould spores tends to occur later in the year in July, August and September. Grass pollen is very light and is spread in the air for many miles so there is little advantage in living in the middle of the city rather than in the country. Only a few particles of pollen on a sensitive nose lining are enough to start an attack. Now in the United Kingdom at various centres, a daily pollen count is done. This is the count of the number of specks of pollen on a jelly covered slide. The results of these tests are broadcast and published in various national newspapers so you are warned not to make a trip in the country when the pollen count is high. A heavy fall of rain may clear the atmosphere temporarily and lower the pollen count which will give some short relief to sufferers.

The symptoms in hay fever are a copious, clear, running discharge from the nose and very often the eyes as well. There are severe bouts of sneezing. The pollen count tends to be high in the morning and this is often when the symptoms are at their worst. They may improve during the day and depending on the time of day at which you see your doctor he may or may not believe that you really have severe hay fever. There is often a blockage of the nose and this may disturb sleep. This in turn produces tiredness, irritability and exhaustion. In some people it also makes them very difficult to live with and uncooperative about treatment for their allergy.

The itching may be of the nose, eyes, ears and soft palate at the back of the mouth. Occasionally the blocking of the nose can cause an infection of the sinuses and then the discharge from the nose will become thicker and may be yellow. This is rare and may mean that the whole problem is a cold and not hay fever. The most serious complication of hay fever is asthma caused by a sensitivity to pollen. This most often comes on during the night. It happens in up to 30% of people with hay fever. Sometimes it is so severe that it is necessary to go into hospital. More often it is just an uncomfortable and unpleasant wheeziness. Hay fever altogether messes up what should be the pleasant part of the year, climate-wise, in the United Kingdom.

Many people with hay fever may have it so mildly that they do not bother to see a doctor. If you have it severely, you would probably see your doctor and he must make a correct diagnosis before he can give effective treatment. A doctor should be aware of the plants and trees in his area causing hay fever and when they pollinate.

The symptoms of hay fever are caused as has been described in an earlier chapter. It usually takes several years of exposure to pollen before you get sensitized and this is probably why it does not occur in young children. Getting sensitized probably depends on an inherited tendency to allergy plus exposure to an irritant such as pollen. The susceptible person develops a special substance in his blood known as reaginic antibody. This clings tightly on to certain cells in the eyes, skin and mucous membrane lining the nose. When the pollen gets into contact with these potentially dangerous cells they break down and histamine is let loose. This has a most dramatic result. The small blood vessels become more permeable and fluid comes out of them leading to the running of eyes and nose. It also causes swelling of the mucous membranes. Cells in the mucous membranes gush out their contents. There is also contraction of smooth muscle which constricts the small airways in the lung and is part of the cause of wheezing if asthma starts. It may be difficult to diagnose hay fever the first year you have it though when it comes back the same time next year the diagnosis is easier. It may help if you keep an accurate diary of the times of the days on which you have the worst symptoms and your doctor can check this against the pollen counts for those days.

There are many centres now in the United Kingdom for investigation and treatment of allergic illnesses and your doctor may send you to one of them. He will do this particularly if you have severe hay fever or if you develop pollen induced asthma. At the centre you will again have to explain your problem and you will be asked about the allergic troubles that you have had such as asthma or eczema and about these illnesses in your family.

When the doctor examines you he may find you have swollen, reddened, runny eyes. Your nose may be blocked and may be running freely. You may be obviously tired and depressed. If he looks up your nose, the mucosal lining will be swollen and paler than normal. In a cold it would be redder than normal. If the doctor examines some of the discharge from your nose under a microscope he will find an increase in one special sort of blood cell called an eosinophil. If the doctor thinks you have hay fever but the discharge from your nose is thick and the mucosa is redder than normal, he will probably arrange for you to have an X-ray to be sure your sinuses are not infected.

The diagnosis will probably be confirmed by skin tests. Small amounts of a solution containing different pollens and mould spores are placed on the skin of your forearm or between your shoulders and the skin is just pricked through these drops. If you are sensitive to any of the pollens tried a red swelling will appear in about ten minutes. In the United States some doctors inject the solution containing pollen into the skin but this is not the usual practice in the United Kingdom because it can cause a serious reaction. There may be false positive reactions and these are usually ignored in the treatment. The important thing is to tie up the results with the times at which you get your hay fever. False negative reactions may be further investigated. Tests can be done called provocative tests in which the suspected substance is sprayed directly on to the nasal mucosa. This should only be done by an expert allergist because it can bring on a serious attack of asthma.

The most serious complication of hay fever is undoubtedly asthma. An infected sinus can be a nuisance but the infection can usually be cleared up with the right drugs. Occasionally nasal polyps may develop but this is more usual in the nasal allergy that is continued all the year round. In children sometimes the swelling round the back of the nose can cause a type of infection in the middle ear called chronic serous otitis media. This can be difficult to treat and can cause deafness. Rarely an urticarial rash can come with hay fever in parts of the skin that have been in contact with grass pollen.

The ideal way of dealing with hay fever is to prevent it happening but this is easier said than done. Living in the middle of a city will not help very much because as has already been explained, grass pollen is very light and is carried for miles in the air. An air-conditioned office helps if the windows are kept closed. Air-conditioned houses are not usually available in the United Kingdom but have been tried in the United States with varying degrees of success.

During the hay fever season it is best to sleep with the bedroom windows shut and drive the car with the windows shut. This helps reduce the pollen you are breathing in. Summer holidays are best taken in early May if you do not have a family to consider. Otherwise take them as late in the school holidays as possible. It is best to avoid walking through long grass at any time and trips into the country during the hay fever season are best avoided. Camping is always better avoided whether in the United Kingdom or elsewhere in Europe. Filters of wet muslin over the open windows do help lower the amount of pollen coming into a room. The ideal way of prevention is a long cruise but for most of us this just is not on.

Treatment can be either locally to the inflamed areas or generally to lower the body's reaction to substances to which it is allergic.

The first treatment tried is usually taking antihistamine drugs. These help counteract the effects of histamine released during the allergic reaction. They are often very effective and probably relieve the symptoms quite adequately in 70–80% of sufferers from hay fever. It may take some trial and error before the best antihistamine drug is found for you. The snag is that the most effective long acting ones can cause drowsiness and some mental confusion. The milder, short acting one may not relieve the symptoms. Sometimes a dose of a long acting antihistamine taken at night will give good relief for 24 hours and the drowsiness wears off during natural sleep. It may be necessary to top this up with a milder, short acting antihistamine after breakfast.

Antihistamine drugs will relieve the itching and the running nose and eyes. They will not deal with the effects of a blocked and possibly infected sinus and they will not deal with the narrowing of the tubes of the lung as occurs in asthma.

Antihistamines should not be taken by epileptics and certain of them should not be taken during pregnancy in case they do harm to the developing foetus. You should never drive a car after taking an antihistamine until you know what effect it will have on you. Antihistamines are less likely to make children drowsy. In fact they may have the opposite effect and make them excitable.

Local treatment can be used for the nose and eyes. Nose drops such as ephedrine drops should be used only for short periods and not more than twice a day. They can damage the lining of the nose and make it more swollen. Steroids can be obtained as a snuff and this can be inhaled up the nose. Some of the steroid will be absorbed into the body through the lining of the nose but not enough to do any damage. This snuff can be very effective. Steroid drops can be used for the eyes and these are more effective and more comfortable to use than antihistamine drops. Steroid or eye drops should not be used for long periods.

If there is asthma with the hay fever, drugs will be necessary to cause widening of the passages in the lung. If the asthma is not severe it can usually be relieved by ephedrine, Franol or Ventolin tablets. If it is severe it may be necessary to give steroids by mouth or by injection.

Steroids should only be given if the hay fever or accompanying asthma is really severe and cannot be controlled in other ways. Recently an injection of a long acting steroid has been tried and been found to be effective in more severe cases of hay fever. The effect lasts for up to a month. In pollen induced asthma, steroids may be given at the beginning in larger doses, gradually reducing the amount to a minimal maintenance dose.

A recently used drug which is good at preventing both hay fever and asthma is disodium cromoglycate, Intal. A spray with it called Rynacrom can be used up the nose to treat the hay fever and capsules of Intal can be taken to prevent asthma. It is very important that you realise this is preventive and to be used all the time during the hay fever season and not just to be used when things are bad.

Desensitizing injections of various sorts have been used

since the beginning of this century. There are various types that can be used but it must first be decided that the inconvenience of the hay fever is more than the inconvenience of repeated injections over several years. In the United Kingdom it is usual to give a course of injections starting about three months before the beginning of the hay fever season. They should be given if the hay fever is getting worse year by year and should also be given if either asthma develops or if the symptoms are severe enough to need steroids by mouth or injection.

There are three types of injection that can be given. The one in water needs 20 to 30 injections. The injections can be given in a mineral oil emulsion and these need only two to three injections. The snag with the latter is the possibility of a severe reaction happening about eight hours after the injection. The third method and now the one most commonly used is alum precipitated extracts. Eight or nine injections of these are necessary. There is no point in going on with injections if there is no improvement after two courses.

These injections are not usually given to children under the age of 5 and between 5 to 12 only if the hay fever is very severe and the child can understand the value of the injections. The injections are not usually given to pregnant women.

Hay fever can make the most enjoyable time of the year into the most miserable for the sufferer. With expert help and treatment it can usually be kept under control so that life is tolerable and there is always the vista of a hay fever free old age.

In many ways allergic rhinitis is similar to hay fever. Allergic rhinitis means a constant or more or less constant state of allergy by the mucous lining of the nose to a number of things. In hay fever, strictly used, the inside of the nose is only allergic to the pollen of grasses but as we have already seen this may be stretched to include other weeds, some trees and moulds. Allergic or perennial rhinitis may in fact include hay fever but the term is used to cover many other allergy inducing things and in some ways it is different from hay fever.

The nose is basically a sensory organ for the appreciation of smell. It also has other functions including warming and cleaning the air that is breathed in by nose breathers. Small particles such as soot, pollen, mould spores and house dust are left on the nasal mucous membrane. The normal mucous membrane has hairs which help these specks move in a downwards direction and clear the nose and it is also helped by the mucous which is normally excreted in moderate amounts by special cells in the mucous membrane. The nasal mucosa is very susceptible to infection and to sensitization to the substances which land on it.

Allergic rhinitis therefore, is not seasonal in the same way as in hay fever. When it occurs there is a running nose, sneezing and headaches. There is also running and itching of the eyes very often. All these symptoms may occur within a few minutes of exposure to the cause of the trouble, for example a cat or a dog. There may be intense running of the nose and sneezing. If the patient is so acutely allergic and if the allergen is house dust there is usually some blockage and running of the nose all the time. Sneezing occurs particularly in the morning.

On examination, the mucosa lining the nose is found to be thickened and boggy in appearance. The colour of it may vary from a dull red to a pearly grey. Very often in allergic rhinitis polyps are present in the nose. These are small bunches of mucosal material and look like minute grapes. They usually grow high up in the nose and hang downwards to cause some blockage of the airways through the nose.

Allergic rhinitis is by definition, caused by certain substances which act as allergens. These may include very commonly, house dust with its content of the house dust mite, the dander of cats, dogs or horses, feathers and cosmetics, particularly face powders. The allergens may also include food particles spread especially to the housewife during the preparation and cooking of food. For men the allergens may include insecticides and wheat flour in those people working with it.

Just to make matters more complicated there is another form of rhinitis called vasomotor rhinitis which is not brought on by allergens in the same way as hay fever or allergic rhinitis. All investigations for allergens are negative including skin tests. The symptoms are the same but they may be brought on by such things as heat or cold or fatigue. They may also be brought on by emotional factors such as anger or even looking forward to something with pleasure. One patient I had always had the symptoms of rhinitis after sexual intercourse. It sometimes comes when a woman is pregnant and disappears again within days or weeks of the end of the pregnancy.

In allergic rhinitis the patient is probably more liable to get his nasal mucosa infected by viruses or bacteria. The swelling of the nasal mucosa makes it particularly liable to infection by viruses and bacteria. The resistance of the normal mucosa to infection depends in part on its acidity. The normal acidity is decreased during the allergy and this causes an increase in the likelihood of getting colds. The increase in infection by viruses will make the patient more prone to colds. This can make the diagnosis very difficult. What looks like an interminable string of colds may in fact be a few colds and an underlying allergic rhinitis. It is very important that this possibility should be considered both in children and adults for those who seem to have an excessive number of colds. Very little can be done about treating a cold but usually quite a lot can be done to treat allergic rhinitis so it is obvious that the possibility should be in the mind of a doctor and of his patient.

In the diagnosis of allergic rhinitis, as in the case of hay fever, it is extremely important for the doctor to take a very careful history. If you suffer from allergic rhinitis it may be a good idea to keep a note of the days during which you have it badly and try to relate it to what you have been doing, with what you have been working and anything you have eaten. Food is not a common allergen in causing allergic rhinitis but some foods can occasionally cause it. The doctor will need to know your occupation and when and where the attacks occur. A housewife who has allergic rhinitis throughout the year is probably allergic to the house dust mite but this can be proved by a further examination.

Aspirins can cause allergic rhinitis so it is important that you tell your doctor of any drugs you are taking. Aspirins are so commonly taken in most developed parts of the world that to many people they are no longer looked on as drugs but an aspirin is a drug. It should only be taken if absolutely necessary and probably the only reason for taking it for a considerable time is in the treatment of rheumatoid arthritis.

It may be necessary for the doctor to find out in which room of the house the rhinitis starts. Some housewives may notice it only when making beds and it can be due to feathers in pillows and eiderdowns. Others may get it in a damp room or cellar and it can be due to moulds. Occasionally it occurs when peeling new potatoes. Usually contact with a cat or dog provokes sneezing and running nose immediately if animal dander is the cause and then it is obvious. It can be caused in the kitchen or bathroom by soap or detergent.

The diagnosis is usually fairly obvious when a really careful history is taken. Allergies can be confirmed by skin testing. This can be done easily and successfully with house dust, animal danders, feathers and many other substances. It should never be tried with aspirin because a very severe reaction with asthma can be caused. A trial of avoiding the offending substances can clinch the diagnosis but in the case of a housewife sensitive to house dust a trial just is not practical unless she has a very unusual amount of help in the house.

The swelling of the nasal mucosa, in allergic rhinitis of the all-the-year-round type, can cause infection of the nasal sinuses. Swelling of the mucosa at the back of the throat can also block the eustachian tube, the small passage that runs between the middle ear and the back of the throat. This can cause infection of the middle ear called otitis media. For some unknown reason, these complicating infections are very much more likely to happen in this type of rhinitis than in seasonal rhinitis or hay fever. The presence of nasal polyps which have already been described can increase the blockage and likelihood of infection of the nasal sinuses. Anybody who has recurrent attacks of nasal sinusitis or chronic sinus trouble should be investigated for underlying allergic rhinitis which could be the cause of the whole trouble.

A do-it-yourself way of treating allergic rhinitis is by using nasal drops which can be brought across the counter in any chemist's shop. These drops are usually the sort that cause vasoconstriction, that is narrowing of the blood vessels of the nasal mucosa. At first, the relief from symptoms is considerable. However, these drops tend to cause a rebound dilatation of the blood vessels when the nasal mucosa gets even more swollen and the patient's symptoms get worse. The tendency can be to use the drops even more frequently and the result is the worsening of the whole condition. It is difficult for a doctor to explain to somebody that he is making himself worse by the use of these drops. This condition where the nasal mucosa is irritated by the prolonged use of nose drops is known as 'rhinitis medicamentosa'. Some drops used over long periods can cause the growth of nasal polyps. It is very inadvisable to use any nose drops except those supplied by your doctor. These will only be prescribed for a very short time. It can be very difficult for a doctor to get a patient to stop using nose drops on which he has become dependent and it may mean the temporary use of steroids to wean him off the drops before better treatment can be started. Antihistamines and sedatives may also be necessary. The condition should be improved in about four or five days.

About a third of people with allergic rhinitis will have or will later develop asthma. Some of these will also have allergic skin disorders such as urticaria. This is the technical word for what is called frequently nettle-rash and which comes on as the result of touching certain things including some plants and highly perfumed soaps or eating certain foods.

In allergic rhinitis the diagnosis can usually be made by a good history and clinched with skin tests. If the nasal secretions or blood are examined in a person with allergic rhinitis it will usually be found that there is an excessive number of eosinophils. These are one of the sorts of white blood cells and are increased in the allergic person.

In the allergic person irritation of the nasal mucous membrane may occur on exposure to irritants which do not come within the definition of allergies. The mucosa is more sensitive and may react more vigorously to such irritants as smoke, fog, or even drinking alcohol.

Hay fever and all-the-year-round rhinitis are very similar in many ways. In their treatment they are different. Once a patient has been found to be allergic to grass or other pollen it is possible to desensitize him but in the case of allergic rhinitis there are many more problems in treatment including the complication such as chronic sinus infection and nasal polyps.

The ideal way of treatment is to find the allergen that is responsible and avoid it. This is much more easily said than done. If a man is found to be sensitive to inhaled wheat flour and he is a miller, it is advisable for him to change his job. If a housewife is found to be sensitive to the house dust mite, she cannot be advised to change her job and the best course is for her to have desensitizing injections combined with drugs to give immediate relief.

Sometimes a member of a family is found to be allergic to the dander of a much loved household pet. Some eminent doctors advise that the pet should be destroyed forthwith. The emotional harm that this may do can far outweigh any benefit derived from such an action. The parent or child can usually be desensitized and this is probably the better thing to do.

When the allergen, or more commonly the allergens, have been found by skin tests and possibly by trials of avoiding the offender, desensitizing injections can be started. These can be begun at any time of year in allergic rhinitis because usually there is repeated or constant exposure to the allergen. Injections are usually given in increasing doses at weekly intervals. Once a satisfactory dosage has been reached, injections can be continued at two to four weekly intervals for a considerable time. This may need to be repeated at yearly intervals, for up to five years when permanent desensitization may be reached. Skin tests should be done every year to check the level of sensitivity.

This sounds rather a heavy penalty to be paid for freedom from sneezes but as many sufferers know, having allergic rhinitis can be a major inconvenience. Without treatment, the outlook is pretty gloomy and the trouble will not usually get better by itself.

Desensitizing injections are the long term and possibly permanent treatment. In the meantime the sufferer will need more immediate relief.

Antihistamines will usually give a good deal of relief. Long acting antihistamines can be given at night which may be sufficient to give relief for 24 hours. Short acting antihistamines can be given during the day but a trial dose should be taken before driving a car or using machinery to check that drowsiness will not be caused.

Steroids can be given for a short time for very severe trouble. They are useful while weaning somebody off nose drops. Steroids can be given by mouth which is usually best avoided. They can also be given locally as drops or snuff. This gives very good relief but should not be continued for long periods because of the risks of absorbing the steroid.

Recently a new preventive has been used. This is disodium cromoglycate. It is used in the nose in the form of Rynacrom. It can be used all the time and in some people is very effective.

If nasal polyps are present it is best to treat the allergy first. The local use of steroids will often make the polyps smaller. Surgery may be necessary to remove the polyps but often their removal, although it helps, will not lessen the need for the continuing treatment for the underlying allergic rhinitis which must be continued.

8 Eczema

❖❖❖❖

Eczema is defined in the Oxford Illustrated Dictionary as inflammation of the skin with redness, soreness and itching papules or vesicles discharging serous fluid. Many doctors, especially in the United States, feel that dermatitis which means inflammation of the skin, or eczema-dermatitis should be used instead of the word eczema. It is not an infective disease of the skin and different sorts of eczema, which is the word most commonly used in the United Kingdom, can be produced either by causes inside the person, endogenous eczema, or causes outside the patient, exogenous eczema. Very often it is a mixture of the two sorts of eczema. The patient has a built-in allergic tendency which he may have inherited from his parents but it is something outside that finally triggers off the eczema.

Probably eczema in babies and eczema which starts off in early adult life are parts of the same diseases but they do have some differences and will be described separately.

In all types of eczema the same main changes take place in the skin. There are cracks in the outer surface of the skin. Some substance is let loose from the damaged skin cells.

This substance causes widening of the very small blood vessels in the skin and an easier passage of fluid out of them. There is then a loss of fluid from these blood vessels. Small vesicles like blisters form and these break, causing the typical oozing of eczema. Crusts also form on the skin as the fluid evaporates. In long-standing or chronic eczema there is thickening and often darkening of the outer layers of the skin.

The look of the skin in eczema is typical. The rash is patchy rather than spotty. There is redness, swelling and oozing in the acute stages but the patient feels itching rather than pain. Normally eczema is not infected with germs but if it does get infected then the patient feels pain rather than itching. Scratching always occurs in eczema and usually you can see the scratch marks. Scratching may well cause infection and then there may be a thick discharge from the skin, red lines along the limb and swelling of the lymph gland as occurs in any acute infection.

The various types of eczema that are described are the allergic eczema which more often starts in small children but can start in adult life. In this type of eczema the skin is usually dry and it is usually associated with other allergies such as asthma and hay fever. This is the type which will be described in greatest detail in this chapter. Another common type of eczema is seborrhoeic eczema which can start at any age and will be described more briefly.

Allergic eczema starts most often in a baby between 3 and 6 months of age but can start at a later stage. The causes are not fully known but it is clear from the family history of allergy in these babies that inheritance plays a part in causing it. There is a family tendency for various parts of the body, including the skin, to be hypersensitive to a number of things from egg whites to emotional upsets. Up to 40% of babies who have eczema in their early years go on to develop asthma or hay fever. More than half the babies with eczema have a family history of other allergies not necessarily eczema.

It is thought that eczema in early months is often due to allergy to various food stuffs. At one time skin testing was done, but in the United Kingdom this has now been abandoned. The diagnosis is made on a good history from the parent's careful observation and on the look of the skin.

In adults who develop eczema for the first time, cause is often emotional, although there may again be evidence of the allergic type of response in other ways. The patient may have had asthma as a child. In babies and small children the cause of eczema is seldom thought to be psychological or emotional, although there may well be psychological results. The mother may be repulsed by the sight of her baby with red raw eczema on him and feel she cannot cuddle him. This can be a great loss for the baby because he needs close, warm parental care, possibly more than a normal baby. The constant itching and disturbed nights may well wear out both the mother and her baby, and the baby may become listless or apathetic or irritable. Part of successful treatment for babies with eczema is to reassure a very anxious mother that the baby is normal, will get better, and needs a great deal of tender loving care.

The diagnosis of allergic eczema is made on the history and appearance of the child. It frequently starts when a breast-fed baby is changed onto cow's milk in the early months. Breast-fed babies get eczema less often than bottle-fed babies. It is no good worrying about eczema if for one good reason or another you are unable to breast-feed your baby, but where there is allergy in the family breast-feeding is much safer.

Another cause in the early months seems to be the introduction of cereal of one sort or another to the diet. It is possible that wheat is the greatest culprit in this direction. It is better to start cereals individually rather than in a mixture. For example, give a plain rice cereal and then a barley one and so on. In this way it is easier to see to which the baby may be allergic. As soon as he reacts to food it must be stopped, but if the eczema does not clear up within a fortnight of stopping the food, food alone is probably not to blame.

Eggs, and particularly egg white, can often cause an allergy. If there is a strong history of allergy in the family it is probably better to advise the parent not to introduce eggs until the baby is a year old. It may be safe to start egg yolk earlier, but not the whites which are most likely to cause an allergy. A baby with a tendency to eczema should not wear wool next to his skin, and silk and nylon should also be avoided. Cotton is the safest material. Both the baby's clothes and bedclothes should be of cotton. His blankets should be washed frequently, and for both his clothes and bedclothes, no detergent or biological powder should be used in washing. Soap is safest for his clothing, and his clothes should be kept very well rinsed.

A baby with eczema should not be bathed too frequently, and no highly scented soaps should be used. Where there is an allergic family history it is probably best to avoid highly scented soap or talcum powder all along. A baby in the acute stages of eczema is best not put in water at all, but cleaned gently with olive oil before other medications are used.

Some authorities advise that with a baby of allergic parents it is best to avoid any sort of chocolate in the first year and orange juice. Vitamin drops are in any case used more frequently now than concentrated fruit juice, and they will do no harm either to the baby's allergy, or indeed to his teeth. It is further suggested that an eczematous, or potentially eczematous baby, should have no pets in the household. This is easier said than done, especially in the United Kingdom where pets play such an important part in so many homes. The best that can be done is probably to keep any pets and the baby apart, and not allow the pet into the room where the baby sleeps.

It is also suggested that for eczematous babies only rubber pillows and mattresses should be used, and both should be covered by dustproof material. No stuffed toys should be allowed near the baby unless filled with foam rubber. This is a good council for the potentially eczematous child, but if a child of a year who is already passionately attached to a teddy develops eczema, it will probably do more harm than good to take it away from him. One always has to remember the emotional elements in the treatment of allergic diseases. The curtains and rugs in the baby's room should be cotton and should be washed frequently.

So much for the prevention of eczema in a baby. If a baby does develop eczema it usually starts on the convex surfaces of his cheeks. These get red, hot and finally come out into small blisters which break and ooze. It may spread to his arms and his legs and is usually found in the fold of the elbows, wrists and behind the knees. This is called flexural eczema. There is always a great deal of itching with this type of eczema and there are normally usually obvious scratch marks and there may be infection.

It is always best, if possible to treat these babies at home, as in hospital they are more likely to pick up some infection which will complicate the eczema. It is vital that the baby should have a reprieve from his itching, both for his sake and for his mother's. Otherwise the whole household can be brought to a stage of despair and depression, and there is obviously likely to be a feeling of rejection against the baby that is causing such an upheaval. This is, of course, only true of the more severe cases. With severe cases the parents, as with so many allergies, have to learn to live with it, and 9 out of 10 of these babies will have outgrown their eczema by the age of 10 years. It is less comforting to tell the parents that up to 40% of the same babies will develop asthma. Sometimes as children they will have asthma or eczema, one getting better as the other gets worse.

The best drugs used for the relief of itching are the antihistamines. These should never be used locally on the affected skin. A cream containing antihistamine has a very real danger of causing added sensitivity which will make the rash worse. The most useful antihistamine for babies is probably Phenergan which can be given as a syrup which many babies seem to enjoy. It is particularly useful at night because it tends to make the baby drowsy which is one of the unpleasant side effects for adults of the antihistamine drugs. In a baby, however, who does not have to go to work, or handle machinery, it is a definite advantage. The baby's nails should be cut very short to stop the scratching.

Sometimes if a mother is very agitated about her baby's state it can do as much good to give the mother a mild tranquilliser as her baby a sedative. If it is thought that the eczema is due to cow's milk and the mother is unable to breast-feed her baby, a preparation of soya beans can be used which does not cause allergic reactions.

Once the itch is brought under control attention can be devoted to the local treatment of the skin condition. 1% hydrocortisone cream is one of the best remedies, but should not be used too freely on too wide an area because of the danger of the baby absorbing the steroids into his body. The ointment should be used very sparingly two or three times a day. It may be advisable if the eczema is very widespread to keep the hydrocortisone ointment for the face and to use a coal tar dressing on the arms and legs.

The itching is so much a part of the eczema that it has even been considered that the basic body fault in eczema is an increased itchiness of the skin. This leads to scratching, and the scratching to eczema. Some would say that this is putting the cart before the horse. Certainly antihistamines, in spite of their name, do not act by opposing histamine at the site of the eczema, but centrally on the brain to decrease the feeling of itchiness in the skin.

Steroids should not be given by mouth to small children because they can slow down the child's growth. If the eczema gets infected the right antibiotic should be given to kill the germs which are grown from the skin.

No baby who has, or who has had eczema, should be vaccinated against smallpox. This can cause a condition called eczema vaccinatum which can be very dangerous indeed. Neither should the baby come in contact with anybody, including his brothers and sisters, who have been vaccinated. Now vaccination against smallpox is no longer recommended routinely in the United Kingdom, this will be less of a problem, but some other countries still demand vaccination, and in this case it will be necessary to give a doctor's letter explaining why the baby cannot be vaccinated. This is usually acceptable.

The other potential danger to a baby with eczema is infection with the virus of herpes simplex. This means that anybody with a cold sore, the common name for the most usual form of herpes simplex, should be kept away from the baby.

Adults with allergic eczema may have kept it from infancy and not grown out of it, or they may develop it for the first time in late adolescence or the twenties. This type of eczema is more likely to be either due to a local irritant such as a metal or a detergent in which case it will be described under the contact dermatitis, or to an emotional cause. It is sometimes found that an emotional upset can bring on an attack of eczema. The adult with eczema is often emotionally unstable and it is very important for a doctor to realise this and to go out of his way to get the patient's confidence, and to give him adequate help and support. If you have had eczema for a considerable time and have seen more than one doctor or skin specialist, you will probably be very critical of the help and treatment you get from a new doctor, so he is really up against quite a difficult problem and you will have to try and put your trust in him.

For mild adult eczema the treatment can be as described for a baby, 1% hydrocortisone cream used sparingly on the face and possibly on the hands, and coal tar used on larger areas of the arms and legs or body. Scratching must be kept under control with antihistamines. A long acting one can be given at night, and if necessary a shorter acting one after breakfast. It is important not to drive a car or use machinery after these drugs until you know what effects they are going to have on you.

For severe eczema in adults, it may be necessary to give steroids by mouth. These are usually effective but there are always some risks attached to the taking of steroids, and your doctor will not prescribe them unless absolutely necessary. A short course is best started with a fairly large dose and tailed off to nil after three weeks or so.

Another type of eczema is seborrhoeic eczema which starts most commonly as cradle cup. The scabs and the remaining skin are oily rather than dry. The rash then usually spreads to behind the ears and all the skin folds. In adults it most commonly affects the scalp. Mild cases are just called dandruff. It may spread to the eyebrows and eyelids. The scalp can be treated daily with a special lotion and shampooed weekly following the putting on of a medicated scalp cream. It is very important in the treatment of seborrhoeic eczema as in all the other sorts of eczema, that you should not indulge in any do-it-yourself treatment, especially creams and lotions. You can also do a lot of harm with many ointments which can be bought over the counter at any chemist. All skin troubles need medical advice, often specialist advice and expert treatment.

Yet another type of eczema is discoid eczema. This arises most often on the skin of the arms and legs and commonly starts in middle age. It can be mistaken for another skin disease called psoriasis, or even for ringworm. Discoid eczema appears in round patches with yellow scales on them. It can best be treated with a steroid cream put on at bedtime and covered with polythene dressing.

A further type of eczema, which is not really of allergic origin, is called gravitational or varicose eczema. It comes on the legs, usually low down, where there has been damage to the deep veins affecting the circulation of the blood back to the heart. It may be helped by bathing in a solution of potassium permanganate. Special bandages may be used from the toes to below the knee and left on for a week at a time.

Other types of eczema occur because of frequent contact with substances that damage the skin and will be described in the chapter on Contact Dermatitis. In diagnosing any eczema, especially in adults, it is very important not to miss any possible diagnosis of contact dermatitis, and a good history from the patient can help in this.

It must be realised with eczema as with all other allergies, there is usually no quick cure. You must remain confident and hopeful that in the end it will clear up but for the immediate future you must live with it. Your doctor will be able to control the itching which makes life so unbearable for the eczema sufferer.

9 Urticaria

It has been reckoned that about 1.5% of the entire population of the United Kingdom see their doctor about this skin condition every year. It is probable that a great many more people than this have urticaria but it is too mild and too rapidly passing for them to see their doctors. Most cases of urticaria are not allergic in origin, but as some quite definitely are a chapter on this condition is being included with other allergies in the present book.

Urticaria is also called hives, or nettle rash. The latter name aptly describes the appearance of urticaria. It is raised, whitish or red spots, often surrounded by a red weal and intensely itchy. In one type of urticaria, papular urticaria, there is as its name implies, a small papule on each patch of urticaria. Because of the intense itchiness there are often scratch marks and there may be in long-standing cases of urticaria some additional infection of the skin. The germs enter through the scratches.

Urticaria is caused by the action of histamine in the deeper layers of the skin which makes the small blood vessels more permeable. Fluid oozes through the blood vessels and causes the localised swelling. It is interesting that in appearance it is very like the sting of a nettle because a nettle sting contains histamine. Urticaria occurs most often in children and tends to come and go. It is in most people a mild condition and will clear up on its own without any treatment. In an attack the severity of the condition waxes and wanes from day to day and also in the course of a day. It is often worse in bed, probably because the warmth in bed dilates the surface blood vessels of the body.

Urticaria can become chronic or long lasting, and be very troublesome indeed to cope with medically, and for the patient to live with. In about 4 out of 5 cases of urticaria the precise cause is never found out although it usually either goes away by itself, or responds well to treatment. It is sometimes difficult to distinguish between these two, although of course the doctor likes to think it has responded to treatment.

One type of urticaria can be serious as well as uncomfortable, but it causes no itchiness. This is angioneurotic oedema, or giant urticaria. It can be caused by drugs, or some food, or bee and wasp stings. Deeper tissues than the skin are involved in this trouble. There can be swelling of the face, particularly of the eyelids. There can also be swelling of the mouth and throat. The swelling of the throat can be severe enough sometimes to cause difficulty in breathing. Joints may also become swollen and painful in giant urticaria. It is not a common condition, but can be very alarming.

The causes of urticaria are very often not known, but sometimes if the patient is very observant it may be known without a doubt. It can be due to something breathed in, drugs swallowed, or be due to pressure, heat or cold. Foods that can cause urticaria or be thought to cause urticaria, are legion. One of the common offenders is fish, especially shellfish. Other offenders are milk, fruit which includes strawberries and citrus fruit such as oranges and lemons. Other foods are pork, chocolate, nuts and eggs.

Substances breathed in which can cause urticaria include cosmetics, pollen of grasses, flowers and trees; feathers, kapok and danders from animal coats. Inhalation from fungi and spores from fungi can also cause urticaria. Contact with the skin of certain things including some plants especially primula and caterpillars can cause urticaria at first where the contact has occurred, but it can become more widespread. Drugs are a frequent cause of urticaria and this will be dealt with more fully in the chapter on Drugs and Allergy. Penicillin is one of the commonest drugs and even in minute doses such as may be found in milk can cause urticaria. So many people take aspirin for one of the numerous anti-pain, anti-cold or anti-fever preparations containing aspirin as a matter of course, this may be overlooked when giving a history. It is an interesting exercise to look in our chemist shop and look at such preparations and their contents and see just how many of them contain aspirin.

Laxatives are another possible cause of urticaria, especially ones containing phenolphthalein. Again, these are taken so casually that they are hardly counted as drugs and can be easily overlooked as the cause of the trouble. The 'pill' can rarely cause urticaria. More common causes are various vaccines or toxoids used for immunisation and also the extracts of antigens used for desensitization. The latter can produce urticaria very rapidly after the injection.

A common type of urticaria is the so-called papular urticaria. The most frequent cause of this trouble is sensitization to the bites of fleas from dogs, cats or birds. This occurs most frequently in children between the ages of 2 and 14 years. In the first years of life the body does not produce the antibodies that cause sensitization and after 14 there seems to be some desensitization from continuing bites. This is unlike the continuing exposure to pollen in hay fever which tends to make the hay fever worse. The bites often occur in a band around the midriff and can also be present on the buttocks and limbs. It is always very difficult to make this diagnosis, not because the doctor does not think of it, but because suggesting to an inhabitant of Great Britain that his pet has fleas, is usually taken more amiss than suggesting that the patient himself had fleas. 'Love me, love my dog and never dare to suggest he has fleas'. This interesting condition will be considered further in Chapter 13 on Pets and Allergy.

Physical factors can cause a non-allergic type of urticaria, either heat, cold or pressure can do it. In heat allergy the ultraviolet rays from the sun or more rarely the infra-red rays can produce an urticarial skin reaction within a matter of minutes of exposure to the sun. There is little that can be done to cope with this condition apart from avoiding exposure. Sometimes a cream that decreases penetration by the sun's rays may help. Your chemist may stock one of these creams, or your doctor will recommend one. In some people who are very sensitive to the sun's rays there may be a more general release of histamine in the body and there can be shivering, a feeling of sickness, or actual sickness, pains in the tummy and diarrhoea.

Cold urticaria is an unusual and not an allergic form of urticaria which will be dealt with more fully in Chapter 16 on Holidays and Allergy. It may be inherited as a dominant trait in which case about half the children of an affected parent will have it, or it may develop at any time of life. In severe forms this rare condition is life threatening. There are ways of testing for its presence and an affected person should be warned against chilling, and especially about the danger of cold showers or swimming in cold water, and that means more or less any of the sea around the United Kingdom. The parts of the skin chilled show an urticarial rash and itch. In some people swallowing ice cold fluid causes swelling of the tongue and throat and can make swallowing and breathing difficult.

Occasionally pressure can cause urticaria. This is also a non-allergic cause and the way in which it happens is not exactly understood. Urticaria can appear on the palm of the hand when a mother has been lugging a heavy shopping basket, or it can appear in the groins and around the waist from pressure with a panti-girdle or under a tight dress belt. This problem never gives any cause for worry, and once it is understood the urticaria can usually be avoided.

It is said that psychological factors can cause urticaria. One authority states that between a quarter and a third of all people with urticaria have, or have had, anxiety, tension, depression or tiredness. It is difficult to see that the incidence of anxiety, tension and tiredness in this group could be any different from that in any group in 20th century people. Apart from scepticism about the emotional factors causing urticaria, one can add the very real emotional results of a constantly itching skin that disturbs tranquillity and rest at all times. Certainly mild sedatives such as Valium and antidepressants do help some people with long-standing urticaria that has failed to clear up with other measures. This may well be the result of helping the patient's general condition, and giving him some relief from a very depressing condition.

It has also been found in one piece of research that urticaria is caused by the addition of preservatives and dyes to food and drink. In Sweden there is a list of foods that are free from dyes and additives. It is a pity that there is not yet any such list available in the United Kingdom. In the same piece of research aspirin sensitivity was tested. Out of 52 patients with chronic or recurrent urticaria it was found that 17 reacted not only to aspirins, but that those who were sensitive to aspirins also reacted to certain berries and fruits, including rhubarb, apple and grapes, and to European red wines and beers.

The worst offenders of the additives were found to be the azo and benzoate preservatives, and tartrazine which is a yellow dye. Without a list, which has been mentioned before, it is impossible to know if one is avoiding these but at least you can look at the ingredients in any packed food and if sodium benzoate or tartrazine is mentioned the food is best avoided. Any highly coloured yellow food or drink, including lemonade is best left alone. Sixteen people with chronic urticaria were kept on a diet free from additives for six months, and 13 out of the 16 remained free from urticaria. With the present increase of health food shops and so called pure food it would be worthwhile for any sufferer from urticaria to experiment with a diet based on these foods and dairy products and keep away from any artificially preserved or coloured foods such as bought biscuits, sweets and drinks.

Foods which are entirely safe for aspirin sensitive people include bread, cereals, sugar, butter, eggs, milk, meat, fish, lettuce, potatoes, salad oil, and preferably water to drink. This would not add up to a very inspiring diet, but would probably be worth trying to keep free from continuous itching. Any patient with urticaria should cut down on drinking coffee and tea. No more tea breaks and coffee after lunch. Many patients with urticaria find that their skin condition is worse after drinking alcohol. This may be because it causes dilatation of the blood vessels in the skin. In any case it is worth adding alcohol to the long and depressing list of blacked foods and drink.

In making a diagnosis of urticaria, taking a careful history with the full cooperation and much patience on the part of doctor and patient is absolutely vital. As has been described in Chapter 2 on the Investigations of Allergies, this is always the most important part in making the diagnosis in any case of allergy. Although under urticaria we have included a number of conditions that are not of allergic origin the fact remains that it is still vitally important to get a really good history if the illness is to be unravelled and any really constructive moves made in its treatment and management. At the present time in 80% of cases of urticaria the cause is never discovered. A lot of these people will get better anyway, but there are some who may have months or years of chronic discomfort to put up with. Some of these as yet undiagnosed cases of urticaria could help themselves by keeping a diary as has been described previously, but in urticaria it needs to be a very full diary indeed. It needs to include foods eaten, places visited, animals touched, occupation at work and at home. It also needs to list down any drugs taken which are prescribed by the doctor or bought over the chemist's counter without a prescription. It is the latter about which we all think so little that may be the elusive cause. As has already been mentioned aspirins and laxatives are particularly likely to be the culprits and both are liberally used throughout the developed world.

In papular urticaria after the first shock to the owner has worn off that his pet may have fleas, it is worth trying to corroborate the diagnosis with the help of a vet. Sometimes fine combing deep in the animal's coat will reveal the culprit, but even if fleas are not found visible to the naked eye, or under the microscope, the animal and his bedding should be liberally and regularly treated with the recommended anti-flea preparation. Papular urticaria in small children should always raise the possibility of an infested animal and it is very gratifying for both the patient and his doctor when a scratchy, irritable child can be cured quite dramatically.

The history should include any emotional factors which may be of importance to the patient. Probably emotional factors alone are never responsible for any allergic condition but sorting out any problems can never do anything but good. There must always be a partnership between the doctor and his patient in the investigation and treatment of an allergic illness, and it should be possible for you to talk freely about any problem whether it is an itchy rash or a marital conflict.

A skin test is rarely of any value unless the urticaria is associated with hay fever and asthma, and seems to be caused by an allergen that is breathed in. Rarely urticaria is due to allergy to the house dust mite, and in this case a skin test may be of value and successful desensitization may be done. In urticaria due to the house dust mite patients characteristically improve when away from their home environment and get worse again on their return. Elimination diets may be tried if there is any certainty that an item of food is the cause, and if it is known within reasonable limits which food is involved. It is very important not to have an elimination diet that is below the level of nutrition that is necessary. Any dieting, unless absolutely necessary, is better avoided in adolescence.

A general physical examination will always be done in urticaria if it is at all troublesome or long lasting. It can be associated with a more severe underlying illness, and obviously this possibility must be ruled out. In chronic urticaria a chest X-ray will probably be done and any other investigations that your doctor may consider necessary. A blood test will usually be done, and the white cells especially examined. In allergic urticaria there will be a slight rise in eosinophils. If there is a large rise in eosinophils, and especially if there is swelling round the eyes infestation with a parasite may be suspected. This can be trichinosis.

In urticaria the blood levels IgE immunoglobulin are not raised, even in cases that are believed to be allergic in origin. This is very different from eczema. Probably less than a quarter of cases of urticaria have an allergic cause. There is a possibility that there is a family history of allergy in a certain proportion of the families of the people with urticaria.

It is necessary in some cases of chronic urticaria for the doctor to get thoroughly acquainted with the patient's work. It may be necessary for the doctor to make enquiries about the process in which his patient plays a part. Some industrial materials such as platinum salts, ammonia, sulphur dioxide, formaldehyde and fumes from acetylene welding can rarely cause urticaria. The urticaria is seldom severe enough or uncontrollable enough to make a patient change his job.

In some people drugs such as morphine, codeine, atropine or pethidine when injected or taken by mouth cause a breaking down of mask cells and a release of histamine. The histamine can cause urticaria.

Dermatographism is an interesting sign which may show in people with urticaria. It is, however, present in about 5% of the whole population. If firm pressure is made on the skin, usually on the back in a line, or the form of writing, in a few minutes a raised white line with a red flare appears. This usually settles in about 20 minutes and disappears, but rarely a more delayed type can occur that takes 6 to 8 hours to appear, and takes 24 to 48 hours to disappear completely. The meaning of this phenomenon is not completely understood.

The general treatment and management of urticaria is often unsatisfactory. It may be difficult to discover the cause and so to eliminate the offending agent. Sometimes this can be done in food allergies, or in papular urticaria when animal fleas can be killed off. More often than not, however, it just is not possible to discover the cause and so treatment must be aimed at damping down the response.

The first drug usually used is an antihistamine. This relieves the itching and rash in about 80% of people, and so is a very satisfactory drug. As always with antihistamines it is necessary to find the best and most effective one with the fewest side effects for that particular person. It just is not possible to predict the reaction and the usual warning must be given that a car should not be driven, or any machinery used until the amount of drowsiness caused by that particular antihistamine is known.

Desensitizing injections are not usually recommended or helpful, but may be done if the allergen is inhaled and the trouble is associated with hay fever and asthma. It may also be done for the house dust mite. Most important desensitization is if urticaria has appeared as part of a serious reaction to wasp or bee stings. This is a very definite indication for desensitization and will be discussed more fully in Chapter 16 on Holidays and Allergy.

Angioneurotic oedema if serious will need urgent medical attention. Artificial respiration may be necessary and a subcutaneous injection of adrenalin. In very severe cases steroids may be necessary by injection.

Local treatment of urticaria is not much help. Probably plain calamine lotion helps as much and does as little harm as anything. A non-scented talcum powder may also help the itch. Antihistamines should be avoided like the plague because of the danger of becoming sensitized to them.

Sedatives may be necessary to help sleep at night if the patient is very itchy. Antidepressants and tranquillisers may be necessary if the patient is very upset or depressed, but this will be discussed more fully in Chapter 15 on Allergy and the Mind.

10 Contact dermatitis

Contact dermatitis must be distinguished from a similar but different sort of dermatitis which may be called irritant dermatitis. Irritant dermatitis is not a sort of allergy and will happen to anybody. Examples of this are the irritation and possibly rashes on the skin which occur after exposure to strong acids and alkalis. There are many other chemicals with which this will happen and when it occurs with normal skin and with everybody, it is not called contact dermatitis.

A sub-division of contact dermatitis is called industrial dermatitis. This is contact dermatitis which its name applies, that occurs at work especially in industry. When diagnosing contact dermatitis it is very important that the doctor decides whether it has started at home or at work because if it is the latter there may be the question of compensation and also the possibility that a change of occupation may be necessary. It may be easier to identify industrial dermatitis if it is known that the patient is handling materials that are likely to cause dermatitis.

In contact dermatitis the sufferer has become sensitized to the stuff that is causing the dermatitis. In most other people the same stuff could be put on their skin and no trouble would appear. There is no reaction of the skin when it first comes in contact with the substance which later causes trouble but repeated or continuous contact over weeks or possibly months can lead to real trouble.

Contact dermatitis is rather like eczema. The main difference is that it occurs first in the area of skin which is in contact with the sensitizing stuff and also that the people in which it occurs are not generally allergic in type. The skin is at first reddened and later small blisters may form. The skin is always itchy and if it is not itchy the doctor should be very wary of making a diagnosis of contact dermatitis. If the dermatitis is of long standing there will very likely be thickening of the skin as occurs in chronic eczema and is known as lichenification. Lichenification means that the skin becomes hareened and leathery as the result of longcontinued irritation.

Contact dermatitis occurs first in the area that has been in contact with the cause of the trouble and this localisation may help in diagnosis as will be explained later. However, the rash may spread to other parts of the body and then there is much more difficulty in making an accurate diagnosis unless the patient has a good memory and can still tell the doctor the exact places where the trouble started.

There is often infection in contact dermatitis because of repeated scratching. Germs are introduced into the angry, weeping skin, and a generalised infection can be a serious and difficult complication to treat.

Contact dermatitis does not usually occur in people with a personal or family history of allergy although with an incidence of allergy of at least 10% in the entire population of the United Kingdom, there are bound, even only by chance, to be some people with contact dermatitis who have a history of allergy. The blood level of the immunoglobulin IgE is not raised in contact dermatitis as it is in allergies such as some cases of asthma and most cases of eczema. Contact dermatitis is a delayed type of hypersensitivity and not an immediate one as occurs in hay fever or some asthma. This delayed type of hypersensitivity may be known as

Type IV hypersensitivity and has been described in Chapter 1 on What Is Allergy. Once a sensitization to some substance is set off, the reaction usually lasts for many years. Sometimes however, a process known as 'hardening' occurs and the sensitization seems to come to a stop. The people can once more be in contact with the substance which previously caused trouble. This 'hardening' is not understood but may be some form of desensitization. In allergies this does not usually occur as for example in hay fever continued expose usually leads to worse hay fever and possibly in the end to pollen asthma.

Contact dermatitis, unlike eczema, is commoner during the middle and later years of life. It is possible for it to occur at an earlier age such as adolescence but it is rare. It does not occur in younger children.

If a rash starts developing on exposed areas of your body such as face, hands or arms, it is important that you see your doctor straight away. It is always much easier for any doctor to make a diagnosis straight away and for the patient to give him an accurate history of how it all began within days, or at most weeks, rather than months. If a rash is left for a long time before a doctor sees it, the patient's memory obviously becomes faulty about the exact way in which the rash started and what seems to have brought it on. If the rash is left untreated by a doctor, the patient is all too likely to try some patent remedy from the chemist's to try and put right what may at first seem to be a trivial skin affair. As has been, and will be said many times in this book, it is never safe to try do-it-yourself remedies. Probably with skins, more damage can be done than with any other condition discussed here. Many creams sold freely and displayed on the chemist's counter contain antihistamines. There are various preparations containing calamine and antihistamine and if the rash is very itchy at first sight this is just the thing. Antihistamines put on the skin are very likely indeed to cause sensitization themselves, and turn a skin condition that might have been treated fairly easily by an expert into a much more serious affair. When the patient finally decides to go for medical advice, the rash has become much more complicated and in addition, the patient may either forget to, or not like to, tell his doctor that he has been treating it himself. An apparently harmless tube of ointment may in itself, seem to be of little importance but if the doctor is told he can help to unravel the diagnostic mystery.

When the doctor first sees somebody with an unexplained rash, which may be contact dermatitis, he will spend time taking a very careful history. If he is in general practice he may know the sufferer well and know what his work is and what his interests are. In this age of increasing mobility the chances are that the doctor, except in a country area, will not know all that much about the patient. He will ask him when the rash started and in exactly what area. He will make very careful enquiries about anything the man did or handled during a day or two before the onset of the rash hence the importance of going to a doctor soon after the rash starts. Months later it will be quite impossible to remember details such as these. The doctor will enquire about work and all the materials that he or she handles at work. The doctor may know that some of these materials are likely to cause contact dermatitis. On the other hand, he may need to visit the work or factory and find out what materials are handled and if possible to have a discussion with the Medical Officer in charge of the workers at the factory. At a large factory this is usually possible but in a small factory or shop, expert assistance may be more difficult to come by.

Having ascertained the job of his patient the doctor will enquire about his home and hobbies. Again it may be necessary to make a visit to the home. The doctor may find that his patient is a keen gardener even of the window-box variety, and has just acquired a new plant that is causing the trouble. Primulas and poison ivy are particularly likely to be the culprits or he may find that his patient is busy building a boat in his back yard and handling some plastic or metal parts that have started the trouble. All in all it takes quiet, persistent detective work at the outset. It is very important that an accurate diagnosis is made at the beginning of this condition because otherwise the months may drag by and the doctor and the patient both get demoralised and the rash no better because the patient is either not having the right treatment or is still in contact with the sensitizing substance.

The next step is a full examination of the patient noticing the exact areas that the rash covers. This combined with a good story of the train of events may be sufficient to give an adequate cause of the rash. In a housewife or hairdresser the rash may be confined to the hands. Then it is relatively easy to find out what the patient is sensitive to taken in conjunction with the history of contacting materials. It may, on the other hand, be just the feet that are involved and may be due to plastic or rubber shoes or the pressure of the shoes or dyed nylon socks. It may be limited to the area of a watch strap or under a place where a certain piece of jewellery is worn.

It is impossible to give a complete list of all the things that can cause contact dermatitis. Almost anything you can think of can cause contact dermatitis in a particular individual but if some clues and examples are given it may be easier to think of the possible cause. It is often impossible for a patient to think of the sensitizing substance at his first visit to the doctor. If he has some idea of what to think about, he may be able to go away and figure out the cause of his problems and go back to his doctor with the correct answer.

The doctor and his patient must think about the possible sensitizing substances at home, at work, handled during the week or weekend or on holiday. Women must think particularly about the things handled in the home and about cosmetics. Most cosmetics can cause contact dermatitis including the so-called hypo-allergenic ones. Admittedly, the latter are less likely to cause trouble but they can. Highly perfumed and darkly coloured cosmetics are generally more liable to cause trouble than say lighter lipsticks and less strongly perfumed talcum powders. A woman may find that she can wear blue eye shadow but not green and one shade of rouge but not another. Allergy to perfumes occurs relatively frequently and will first show itself by the site in which it appears although it may be absorbed by a watch strap if perfume is put on a wrist. Subsequently the watch strap will be held responsible. Generally the site of the original rash will give the clue about cosmetic sensitivity.

Hair dyes, home permanent waving solutions and anti-dandruff lotions are all commonly used and may cause contact dermatitis both on the head where they are used and on the hands which are exposed to these solutions. In the mouth, dental fillings or plates or other appliances can all cause sensitization. Toothpaste can do it and also some soaps and bath essences. One form of contact dermatitis in women can cause some confusion and in recent years has produced a considerable amount of correspondence in the medical journals. This is caused by tights and occurs in the area between the legs and the genitalia. It is not known for certain whether it is dye from the tights brought out by perspiration or the remains of detergent left after washing the tights again brought into close contact with the skin in that area.

Housewives' hands can be a problem. Most housewives, especially those with young children, have wet hands from washing clothes or washing dishes for a fair part of each day. It is possible, but not proved, detergent and biological powders can produce sensitization or they may affect the skin and soften it up for sensitization by other substances such as hand cream. The affected housewife may start wearing rubber or plastic gloves only to find that her hands get worse. This may be because some washing-up water has got inside the gloves or that the hands have become sensitized to the materials of which the gloves are made.

Metal objects made with nickel or chrome can cause trouble. Boys who ride bicycles holding the metal part of the handlebars instead of the grip, can get contact dermatitis of the hands. Men who paint their houses run the risk of sensitization to paint or to turpentine. Plastic repair kits can be responsible. At work, many chemicals and other substances can be responsible. Lanolin is a common ingredient of cosmetics and medically used ointments, and was always thought to be very safe, is now known to be responsible for some cases of sensitization. Lanolin is also present in many shampoos, shaving creams and soaps. In one series of people investigated for contact dermatitis, it was found that 7.4% were sensitive to lanolin. It used to be found that people had negative patch tests to lanolin but now an improved product has been produced for patch testing. The considerable sensitizing possibilities of lanolin have been confirmed. The present product used is 30% wool alcohols in a mixture of olive oil and petroleum jelly because lanolin is made from sheeps' wool wax. It helps if the patch test is done on normal skin near the area of skin that is affected.

Contact dermatitis can occur as the result of treatment either of the do-it-yourself variety as mentioned before, or in the course of medical treatment. Some antibiotics, antihistamines and anaesthetics all used locally on the skin, can cause contact dermatitis. It can occur in the course of other skin conditions such as athlete's foot for which strong medications are being used on the skin.

It is very important that if at all possible the responsible substance should be discovered before any treatment is started. Contact dermatitis is a nuisance rather than a threat to life and if it is allowed to continue unchecked, it can last for many months or years. It can lead to months in hospital, possibly years off work and a very dreary and depressing time for the sufferer. The time spent on good detective work is well rewarded.

If the history and examination give clues as to the cause, selective patch testing can be done on the skin with the suspected substances. This procedure has been described in Chapter 2 on the Investigation of Allergies. If no real clue has been gleaned from the history and examination, a battery of about twenty substances likely to produce contact dermatitis can be used. This is not a very scientific approach and is less likely to give a clear-cut answer than if the substance can be suspected from the history and examination.

The best treatment for contact dermatitis is to avoid the offending substance and this is why it is so important to be sure of the cause of the skin rash. For men it may mean changing their occupation and this is never advised lightly. A housewife may need to change from using detergents or biological powders to pure soap. If she wears rubber or plastic gloves she should be advised to wear a pair of thin, white cotton gloves inside and to avoid getting liquid inside the gloves. A woman may know a cosmetic that causes trouble and can avoid it. She should be advised to use less highly scented and less darkly coloured cosmetics. It is possible to get a list of so-called hypo-allergenic cosmetics from any chemist who sells cosmetics. These are less likely to cause trouble but all reliable manufacturers of cosmetics in the United Kingdom avoid using substances in their cosmetics that are likely to cause trouble.

Desensitizing injections rarely, or never have any beneficial effect in contact dermatitis and are not normally used.

If, when first seen by the doctor, the skin is red, raw and weeping, it is usual to use a wet dressing. This can be any bland fluid such as weak salt solution or potassium permanganate. Ointments and creams are not used until the skin has dried up. The weeping areas should be kept covered by frequently changed wet dressings. Once the area is dry, various preparations can be used. Old fashioned remedies such as Lassar's Paste are still used sometimes but because they are messy there is an increasing use of steroid containing ointments and creams. Sometimes, once a sensitizing substance has been avoided these steroid containing preparations can clear the skin up like magic and this is very pleasing both for you and your doctor.

If there is already infection of the skin when seen by the doctor, antibiotics will probably be used. These should be taken by mouth and not used locally on the skin because of the danger of further sensitization.

Antihistamines are the drugs most useful in helping the itch. At night a long acting antihistamine with very drowsy-making side effects, can be useful in relieving the itch and helping sleep. During the day trial and error will find the antihistamine that most helps the itch and has fewest side effects. As in any treatment with antihistamines, the patient must be warned not to drive a car or use machinery until he is sure what effects the particular antihistamine in use will have on him. Calamine lotion can be used safely on the skin to help the itch but beware of calamine preparations that contain an antihistamine.

If the dermatitis is very severe when first seen, bed rest at home or even in hospital may be necessary. Sedatives and tranquillisers may be used to help the patient to rest. A short course of steroids may be given by mouth but these are discontinued as soon as the patient's condition begins to improve.

It must be stressed that by far the most important part of treatment depends on discovery of the offending substance and getting it out of the patient's immediate environment. Once that is done the rest of the treatment is relatively easy and the patient must be warned that once cured he should continue to avoid whatever was the cause of all the trouble.

11 The gut and allergy

✧✧✧

Allergy to food is probably a fairly common business, but in most cases it may be so mild that a person does not see his doctor. Doctors therefore only see the more severe forms of this particular allergy, or the more puzzling ones.

Allergy can develop to a wide variety of foods. It can be broadly divided into an immediate type of allergic reaction and a delayed type of allergic reaction. It is probable that the immediate type of reaction is caused by the absorption from the gut of partially digested, or undigested food particles. The delayed type of allergic reaction, which may take 24 hours or so to develop, is probably caused by the ingestion of the breakdown products of digestion. The gut of infants is more easily permeated by undigested or partially digested food particles, and they are particularly likely to develop the immediate type of food allergy.

Allergies to food usually occur in people who are in general of the atopic or allergy prone type. Very often in the same patient there are other allergies including asthma, hayfever or allergic rhinitis. Food which is ingested through the gut acts as an allergen and can cause trouble in more or less any part of the body that has blood vessels, mucous membranes, or smooth muscle—that is muscle such as muscle of the gut that is not under the control of the patient. The type of reactions which can be produced by food allergy are therefore legion.

If somebody suspects a food allergy either in herself or in one of her children, she may not see a doctor. If the symptoms are mild, perhaps vomiting after eating certain food in large quantity, the situation may well be obvious and the doctor will not be consulted. Probably doctors as a whole are not aware of the extent of food allergy in the population because they are not seen about the majority of cases. This may either be because the symptoms are so mild, or because the type of illness is not suspected by the sufferer; he may just say he has a weak tummy. If the symptoms are at all severe, especially if their cause is not obvious, the patient will probably see his doctor. It is then up to the doctor to try and unravel the problem and supply what help he can.

The first essential to be undertaken by you and your doctor is a really good history. This is important in all allergies, but especially important in a suspected food allergy. You may already know what food brings on your symptoms and be able to tell your doctor all the answers. It is more likely that you will both have to put your thinking caps on to unravel the problem. The immediate type of allergic reaction to food is always more easily diagnosed than the delayed type. You may know that within minutes of eating a fair helping of a food such as milk, eggs, or a lot of other things, you may come out in an itchy rash or start being sick. The delayed type of allergy is obviously much more difficult to pin down because of the long interval between eating the food and the onset of symptoms.

It may be helpful if after your first visit to the doctor you keep a diary of all foods eaten and the time of onset of your symptoms. Many foods can cause allergic troubles, but amongst the commonest are milk, eggs, fish, especially shellfish, pork, nuts, chocolate, oranges and strawberries. If symptoms only occur every few months there is no point in keeping a regular diary. It will probably be sufficient when an attack occurs to write down in retrospect all the foods eaten during the previous two days.

What is called an elimination diet may be tried if either the attacks are frequent or if there is a chronic problem such as urticaria. This is eating a diet without the suspected food for two or three weeks. If there is no benefit after two or three weeks, the diet should be abandoned. Only one food should be eliminated at a time, and if it is a vital food stuff, such as milk, this should be tried with caution, especially in a child. It is very important not to eliminate a number of foods without good cause because it is very easy to cause food faddism in this way, and in the long run cause the patient far more anxiety and possibly a deficient diet.

Skin tests are of very doubtful value in food allergy. There may be positive results in the immediate type of food allergy. In the delayed type of food allergies skin testing is extremely unreliable. Doubtfully positive skin tests should not influence treatment. There will probably be no good result in leaving out these foods from the diet. As in elimination diets it is all too easy to start off food faddism and possibly a deficient diet.

There are some times hidden sauces of allergen in the food. This can be milk or wheat cereal. These may occur in extremely small quantities in many food stuffs and may not be suspected to be present by either the doctor or his patient. Penicillin is sometimes present to improve the growth of some animals. Minute quantities of this may get through to the human gut and be responsible for an elusive food allergy.

Allergies in infants can be very worrying for a mother because the infant may fail to thrive. The allergy may be to the protein in cow's milk and may start after changing from breast to bottle feeding. There are many causes of vomiting and diarrhoea in an infant, and allergy is not a common one. Probably the commonest cause is just being a 'sicky' baby which is possibly connected with a weak valve between the lower part of the oesophagus and the stomach. The latter type of sickness usually clears up by itself and the baby nearly always thrives well.

In allergy to cow's milk in the infant, there is usually

vomiting and often diarrhoea. Eczema may develop, it usually starts off on the face and often around the mouth. The infant may fail to gain weight and he may also have a great deal of colic in his tummy. Babies can also be sensitive to eggs and to wheat cereal. Sometimes a baby will refuse food containing these, and if made to take it he may be sick or get swelling round his lips.

Food allergy in infants can be a problem to diagnose. Milk allergy has to be distinguished from a failure of enzymes to digest the milk. If milk allergy is finally considered to be the diagnosis, it should be treated by removing milk from the diet. A product containing soya beans can be substituted. This may only need to be done for a limited time, because as the baby gets older he may be able to tolerate cow's milk. It should be given in small quantities at first and it is better to start with either evaporated milk or cow's milk that has been boiled gently for ten minutes. The outlook for a baby with cow's milk allergy is very good, and he will almost certainly outgrow his trouble.

Food allergy in adults can show itself in many forms, although some of those described are so vague as to be confused with almost any form of chronic ill health including chronic anxiety. In chronic anxiety it is important that food is not blamed because otherwise the anxiety may be made worse, and the real cause of the ill health may be further hidden. Severe reactions to food can include anaphylactic shock and angioneurotic oedema with blocking of the air passages. These very acute forms of gut allergy need to be diagnosed and the cause found so that the food responsible may be avoided in future. It needs to be stressed that severe reactions are very rare indeed.

Angioneurotic oedema occurring as a result of food allergy in adults may be mild and show itself with some swelling of the mouth and lips, often urticaria, mild joint pains, and a general feeling of illness. In severe cases, which are very rare, there may be actual swelling of the joints and swelling of the tongue and throat, causing difficulty in breathing. This is a medical emergency and a doctor must be found at once.

Another medical emergency is anaphylactic shock which

again is very rare indeed. In a sensitive person it can occur after eating shellfish. There is a quick reaction with a feeling of faintness and there may be acute asthma. The patient is very shocked and pale with a quick pulse and breathing may be difficult. The patient should be taken to a hospital, or a doctor found, whichever is quicker.

In less severe cases there may be general symptoms of an upset gut. These can include vomiting, diarrhoea, severe colic or a milder feeling of discomfort and blown-upness. In cases which are confined to symptoms in the gut, obviously the doctor has to rule out many causes of pain in the belly and vomiting, such as appendicitis or a blockage somewhere, before he can begin to think about allergy. If there is an appendicitis, obviously this needs urgent surgical treatment, while if the trouble is allergic there is no emergency and it can be investigated at leisure. It will usually be after several attacks that the right diagnosis will be made.

In most cases of gut allergy in adults, eosinophilia may be present in the mucosal lining of the bowel if it is examined microscopically. There may also be an increased number of eosinophils in the blood. In a baby with cow's milk allergy there may be a marked reduction of the proteins globulin and albumin in the blood. All these findings are very variable and the most important finding in taking the history is the eating of a certain food regularly before the start of the illness.

In the treatment of food allergy the aim should be to get the offending food out of the patient's diet. This may be easy if it is something such as strawberries, pork or shellfish which can be well avoided. It may be difficult if it is milk, eggs or wheat cereal because they are present in so many foods and also because they form a vital part of the human diet. No articles of diet should be left out unless there is very strong evidence that it is the culprit.

It may be found that a food may be tolerated if taken in small quantities and rarely. A food stuff may cause trouble if it is taken every day, but not if it is only taken once a week. Also cooking may help reduce the allergic properties of a food. Uncooked foods are much more likely to cause allergies than cooked food. After a certain food has been left out of a diet for several months it may be tried again in small quantities because sometimes the sensitivity may have got less. This should not be done with such foods as strawberries that have caused an anaphylactic reaction. They are better avoided altogether for good because the risk of another reaction is always possible and strawberries may be agreeable but are not in any way a necessary food.

Antihistamines or in the case of colic, gut antispasmodics, may help treat the symptoms of gut allergy. Desensitization by injections is of no value. Medical emergencies, such as anaphylactic shock, need immediate medical attention because only a doctor can treat such a condition adequately. The most important treatment, however, is avoiding the food that causes the trouble and this may only be necessary for a limited time.

12 Drugs and allergy

❖❖❖

Reactions to drugs are more common all the time because of the increasing use of drugs by doctors and patients. Not all of the drugs that a patient takes are prescribed by a doctor. It is very usual for people to take pain killers, most commonly aspirins, or laxatives, without asking their doctor. Also substances are taken in some food and drinks without their presence being known. Penicillin may be present in very small amounts in meat and milk. Quinine is present also in small amounts in tonic water and bitter lemon drinks. When an investigation is going on into a suspected drug allergy these, what one might call secret sources of drugs, must be kept in mind.

In one investigation into drug allergies in the United States, it was found that 15% of patients in a teaching hospital had reactions to the drugs which had been prescribed for them. Not all of these reactions were allergic, but nevertheless it can be seen that reaction to drugs is a considerable problem. Both in the United Kingdom and in the United States all drug reactions are supposed to be reported to a special committee. This committee acts as watchdog on all drugs used and their ill effects. Many mild ill effects by drugs go unreported both by patients to their doctors, and by doctors to the committee. It is obvious that the known reactions to drugs are not the true picture, and the true picture would in fact show up many more ill effects than are at present known.

Reactions to a very high dose of a drug can occur and these should be called toxic reactions. Moderate or even small doses of a drug can be taken, but because either the liver or kidneys are not working properly, the patient is unable or slow to excrete the drug. This will lead to a build-up of the drug in the patient's tissues and quite possibly to a toxic reaction.

The term 'drug allergy' should be kept for those instances when there is a known type of allergic reaction between the drug and the cells of the patient. In many cases it is assumed that there is an allergic reaction, but it is not possible to prove it. Probably about a quarter of all the drug reactions are allergic in character. The allergy may be a Type I allergic reaction. This is an immediate reaction and occurs in such types of drug allergy as urticaria or anaphylactic shock. It may also be a Type IV allergic reaction as occurs in contact dermatitis. Drugs are most likely to cause an allergic reaction when put locally on the skin, and least likely to cause an allergic reaction when taken by mouth. Injected drugs come between those put on the skin and those taken by mouth.

Usually there is a previous history of taking the drug before an allergic reaction occurs. The drug may have been taken by mouth previously and later when given by injection causes an allergic reaction. The drug by mouth has then acted by sensitizing the patient's cells. The type of drug may affect the likelihood of an allergic reaction. Some drugs are very unlikely indeed to cause an allergic reaction, but drugs such as penicillin cause a great number of allergic reactions.

Adults are more likely than children to suffer from allergic reactions to drugs. Penicillin can be used repeatedly for infections in children, and allergic reactions are very rare. There is some evidence that people who have an allergic history or who in other words may be called atopic, are more likely to get drug reactions of the allergic type. People who are allergic to one drug are possibly more likely to become allergic to other drugs. Especially when seeing a new doctor if you are away from home or on holiday when you get ill, you should tell him about any allergic reactions to drugs which you have had before he prescribes for you.

The amount of drug given, and the length of the treatment, are not closely connected to the likelihood of having an allergic reaction. An exception may be large doses of penicillin, particularly if given by injection. Allergic reactions may be commoner if repeated short courses of a drug are given with a gap between. If you become allergic to a drug you are likely to remain allergic to it even in very small amounts.

In desensitizing injections and in some immunisations, the active substance has something added to it called an adjuvent. This adjuvent increases the chance of an allergic reaction to the injection. The advantages of having an adjuvent in desensitizing injections are that fewer injections may be necessary to have the desired effect. Some people are particularly likely to be allergic to immunisations where the active substance has been grown on a chick embryo. These are all problems that your doctor has to think about when recommending a course of treatment.

Any type of allergy can be produced by drugs, including an anaphylactic reaction, serum sickness, urticaria, asthma, allergic rhinitis, contact dermatitis. Anaphylactic reactions are the most severe and the most frightening reactions which can be caused by drugs. They usually follow an injection but can rarely occur after a drug is given by mouth when the reaction will take longer to develop. There will be the usual picture of feeling unwell, possibly collapse, raised pulse rate, and being pale and sweaty. Such a reaction may occur after an injection of penicillin, or after a desensitizing injection with an adjuvent. When giving short courses of such desensitizing injections your doctor will possibly ask you to stay around for twenty minutes or so. If you then have a serious reaction it can be treated immediately. Usually an anaphylactic reaction occurs when it is not the first time that the body has met that particular antigen. Occasionally such a reaction can occur on the first occasion that the body meets the antigen. In the latter case the patient is usually an allergic type and has raised levels of IgE immunoglobulin in his blood. There is usually also a history of asthma or hay fever.

When diagnosing a drug allergy a number of factors have to be taken into account to avoid blaming a drug unjustly. If a drug, or drugs, are blamed without due cause they may be stopped and this may seriously interfere with a patient's treatment. Also if one particular drug is held responsible it will be banned for all time, and this may upset future treatment for what could be a serious illness. It is very difficult to be sure when a drug is responsible for an allergic reaction. The history needs to be taken into account, and the possibility of a skin reaction occurring as part of the illness considered. In the case of an injection given in a well person an allergic reaction may be obvious. In the case of a reaction occurring in the course of treatment for an illness with fever, it may be far more elusive. If penicillin is responsible and is being given by mouth the reaction may not occur until about the tenth day of treatment. The diagnosis has to be based on probabilities, and not on scientific facts which can make it very difficult indeed. A rash may occur anyway in the course of the illness. The possibilities of the drug acting as an allergen, and the patient acting in an allergic way, have to be weighed up before any decision can be made. Skin tests for hypersensitivity to a drug are of little value.

It can be said that drugs being taken are blamed too often by both the patient and his doctor when a rash appears. If the drug is being used locally on the skin for an already existing rash which becomes rapidly worse after starting treatment, the conclusions may be different. A lot has been learnt in recent years about skin allergies, and many preparations formerly in frequent use on the skin have fallen out of favour. These include all creams and ointments containing penicillin and sulphonamides, local anaesthetics and antihistamines. There is a further tendency to use fewer preparations on the skin which have any antibiotic in them as has been mentioned in Chapter 10 on Contact Dermatitis. Even lanolin as a base for creams, which was formerly thought to be very safe, is now suspect. It is getting to the point where it is almost better to advise scratching for an itchy skin rather than putting anything on it. The two so far absolutely safe things to put on the skin are a weak solution of salt in water, or simple calamine lotion.

Aspirin, and the enormous number of aspirin containing compounds, are the most commonly used drugs in the world. Many pain-killers, cold cures, and anti-fever medicines or tablets contain aspirin. Compounds related to aspirin are in some toothpastes, mouth-washes, childrens' teething powders and in food preservatives. Aspirins are so commonly taken that you may not think of telling your doctor that you have had some when consulting him about an apparently unrelated problem. Aspirins can cause urticaria, but their most worrying effect is causing an attack of asthma in an already asthmatic patient.

If somebody with asthma finds that aspirin makes the asthma worse he should beware of other pain-killers because they may have the same effect. Other responsible pain-killers include paracetemol and indomethecin which is commonly used for rheumatic conditions. The only really safe way for an aspirin sensitive patient with asthma is to avoid all pain-killers unless prescribed by a doctor for severe pain.

Penicillin is responsible for nearly three-quarters of all allergic reactions to drugs, but oddly enough it is quite a safe drug. The reason why it is responsible for so many allergic reactions is the incredible frequency with which it is used. Many patients manage to con their doctors into giving them a course of penicillin tablets for a cold which would get better on its own anyhow. Penicillin should not be used for trivial illnesses and should not be asked for or prescribed unless it is really necessary. There are, of course, many instances when a doctor may consider it necessary such as an acute attack of bronchitis or an early inflammation of the middle ear. If a doctor prescribes it the patient should certainly take it.

Allergic reactions to penicillin occur in between 1 and

10% of people taking it. Penicillin is no longer usually used on the skin which was the most common way of causing an allergy. Giving penicillin by mouth is the safest way, and by injection a little less safe. It has been estimated in the United States that .1% of people having an injection of penicillin get an anaphylactic reaction. If a person reacts to one type of penicillin, for example ampicillin, it is possible that he will react to other types of penicillin and they should be avoided. Your doctor will certainly have a note of it if you have had an allergic reaction to penicillin, and you should tell any other doctor who treats you about it.

An allergy to sunlight can appear in some people on certain drugs. The allergy may show itself at first in a socially acceptable fashion by causing a quick suntan. Later however the exposure to sun can cause an eczematous rash or urticaria. Many drugs will do this including the tetracyclines, some tranquillisers, sulphonamides and some diuretics. Diuretics are tablets which help get fluid out of the body.

No doubt as medicine progresses still further and more and more drugs are introduced there will be more allergic reactions to them. It will be a major advance when it is possible to pinpoint the drug that is responsible for a possibly allergic reaction.

13 Pets and allergy

❖❖❖

It is important to stress just how important a part pets play in the lives of many families in the United Kingdom. Possibly more than in any other part of the world a pet becomes part of the family. This has to be said for two reasons. The first is the intimacy with which many people live with their pets. Contact may be close and frequent and this may increase the part the pet can play in the production or continuation of an allergy. It is firmly said by the medical profession that very close contact with animals should not be encouraged for a number of health reasons. Yet even in families quite responsible about hygiene in other ways pets are allowed in bed and a dog licking a child's or an adult's face is not frowned upon. There is always plenty of petting and stroking.

The second reason why it is important to say that a pet becomes part of the family is because this affects the advice given to a family when a pet is found to be the cause of an allergy, particularly asthma in a child. It is said categorically by many authorities that of course the pet must be disposed of. I feel that this advice without qualification is just not acceptable. Those who recommend immediate removal and possibly destruction of the pet have left out of account the intimacy that can grow up between even quite a small child and a family cat or dog. The animal can be part of his family and a loved and loving companion. The removal of this part of the child's security may do him more emotional harm than allergic good. It may be possible to send the pet for a holiday to friends or to kennels and when the child has accepted the idea and is not pining a more permanent arrangement may be sought. While the animal is on holiday there is always the possibility of the return and a child may be more willing to accept this situation. Anybody who can say or write that a pet should be destroyed without further ado just does not understand the workings of probably the majority of families in the United Kingdom. If pets were not so common and so adored I doubt if the phrase 'love me, love my dog', would have become part of the vocabulary.

In an allergic family it is probably better to avoid the acquisition of pets even before the arrival of children. Pets, particularly cats, are frequently the cause of allergic problems, and if the family has never grown accustomed to having a pet around they can avoid the trauma of having to dispose of one. Remembering that the children of allergic parents are very likely to have an allergy it is probably sound preventive action to avoid the addition of pets to the household.

Probably the most serious allergy for which a pet can be responsible in asthma. It is the dander from an animal's fur that is the culprit. Cats are the most common offenders and even a short-haired cat can produce enough dander to cause trouble. Many animal's dander can be responsible for allergy and these include dogs, horses, goats, cattle, hamsters, rabbits and hedgehogs. If it is suspected that an animal is responsible and can be sent on holiday for two or three months further investigations can be carried out. Skin tests can be very helpful. A patient may only be allergic to his particular animal or breed of animals. On the other hand he can be allergic to a wide range of related breeds of his animals. It is best to get an extract of the dander of the particular animal suspected and make a skin test with that.

It is possible that allergy to animals may not be confined to pets but be part of an occupational allergy. Farmers may become sensitive to their cattle or sheep. A pet shop owner may become sensitive to any one of a number of animals. In these days the range of pets sold is very great. A furrier may become sensitive to some of the pelts he works with. A zoo keeper may become sensitive to one of his charges or a worker in a circus may become sensitized to some animal performer. The range is wide. In these cases the diagnosis must be made with certainty before any steps are taken. Skin tests to the dander of the suspected animals or animal, should be done after the worker has been away from them for several weeks. If it is proved that he is sensitive it is usual to attempt a course of desensitizing injections. In the case of asthma the possibility of a severe reaction during desensitization is always present, and this course would only be taken in an attempt to prevent the sufferer having to change his job. If all else fails, including of course routine treatment for the particular allergy, it may be necessary to suggest a change of occupation.

A change of occupation is never suggested until absolutely all else has failed because especially in the case of a middle-aged man without other experience or qualifications it may be extremely difficult for him to find an alternative method of earning his own and probably his family's living. The government does run retraining schemes for men and women of all ages and with all types of disability. One of these schemes should be considered if treatment for an allergy to animals has failed, and the sufferer needs another way of earning his living.

A pet that is responsible for causing attacks of asthma does not necessarily live in the owner's house. It may be a weekly contact and in this case it is very difficult to track the cause down. If it is impossible to avoid the animal in somebody else's house and if the contact is frequent, then it may be possible to take preventive action in the form of medicine before the contact. If the pet is in your own home and it is decided to send him for a holiday while the allergy is investigated, it is important that the dander from his coat, and it is most often a cat's coat, should be thoroughly removed from the house. This means moving out the bed and bedding of the animal, and thoroughly vacuuming any chairs, carpets or rugs where he could have been. This cleaning has to be very thorough to be effective.

Somebody may have contact with an animal for a long time before he becomes sensitive to it. If this sensitivity starts while the patient is having a course of desensitizing injections against another and quite different antigen, it may upset the whole course of treatment. The possibility of a new allergy always has to be borne in mind when there is an increase in symptoms during a course of desensitization. It is true to say that in general pets and allergies do not mix well, but in general in the United Kingdom they just have to rub along in the best way that can be managed. Even after an animal has been removed from the house and thorough cleaning has been done, it is possible that minute particles of dander can remain in the house dust. Although allergy to pets is not seasonal, the movement of dust may be increased and the allergy worsened when the central heating is turned on for the colder weather.

It is possible to have an allergy to horsehair in the upholstery of chair or bed. Also in the case of the rich who can afford such luxuries it is possible to become sensitive to animal's hair used in fabrics such as mohair, cashmere or alpaca.

A relatively common skin problem caused by an allergy connected with pets is papular urticaria. This has also been discussed in Chapter 9 on Urticaria. In one survey in a rural area of Cornwall it was found that one in twenty of all referrals to the skin specialist was caused by this condition. It is an allergy to the fleas on a pet. Not many owners of pets like to admit that their pet could have fleas. Sometimes it seems it might be less complicated to suggest that the owner had fleas rather than his pet. It is particularly difficult to diagnose when it is caused by occasional contact with an animal not owned by the patient's family as it is even more complicated to suggest that the neighbour's pet has fleas.

Papular urticaria can occur in adults or children. It is more common in children and seems to reach a peak between the ages of two and fourteen years. The rash starts as small red spots and is extremely itchy. The spots become small raised weals. There is usually a lot of scratching and as a result there may be some infection of the skin. The patient most often gets medical help between the tenth and fourteenth day of the rash. If the rash has been there for a considerable time there is likely to be thickening and cracking of the skin and there may be darkening in the colour of the skin. Although this allergy is so common it is very often not diagnosed at once by a general practitioner or even by a skin specialist.

It is always very difficult to explain why one member of a family can be affected in this way by an infested animal and not the whole family. It appears that some people have skins that are repellant to all insect attacks. Some people are attacked but do not produce an allergic type of rash, and the sufferers are the ones that both get attacked and do produce an allergic form of rash. This question of only one member of the family having the rash usually comes up when the doctor investigating the problem enquires about either family pets, or pets with which the patient may have had any contact.

The fleas are very small and transparent and are just visible to the naked eye although very difficult to spot. They are very unlikely to have been noticed by the pet's owner and even if a vet is asked to examine the animal it is quite possible that he will miss them. In a case of papular urticaria the suspected pet should be stood in the middle of a large sheet of brown paper and groomed vigorously. Even if nothing is visible to the eye the brown paper should be carefully folded and sealed thoroughly with sellotape. It should be sent for microscopic examination. In one series of pets which were in contact with patients who had papular urticaria 58.3% of dogs, and 70% of cats were found to be infested.

The rash occurs most commonly on the outer parts of the arms and legs, although it can also appear round the middle of the tummy. It is always intensely itchy. The rash usually comes out in new batches every few days and for some reason is most likely to start in the Autumn between the months of August and October.

Fleas can occur on other pets as well as cats and dogs and can cause the rash. Other pets include hamsters, rats and mice, hedgehogs and rabbits. The rash always has to be distinguished from scabies. Scabies on a dog can be caught by a human and can produce an extremely itchy rash but without the typical marks of the burrows seen in human scabies.

In any patient with papular urticaria the infestation of an animal contact must, if at all possible, be ruled out. If this is not done and contact continues all treatment is likely to fail. Once a diagnosis has been made there are two lines of treatment to be carried out. The first is of the animal and this treatment should be supervised by a vet. The second is of the patient. The animal is usually treated four or five times with an anti-flea powder. All the animal's bedding should also be treated with the powder. In the case of rodents or rabbits the old litter should be burnt and replaced with new litter each time the animal is treated. All the soft furnishings in the house with which the animal has come in contact should also be treated with the anti-flea powder. The powder should be left for twenty four hours and then removed with a vacuum cleaner.

The patient should be treated with a cream or lotion to stop the irritation, but not one containing antihistamine or local anaesthetic. For a child simple calamine can be quite effective and is quite safe. An antihistamine tablet or syrup given at night can stop the itch and help sleep at the same time. The rash will clear up by itself once contact with the infested animal is stopped.

Another type of allergy to animals can occur in bee keepers. If a bee keeper gets sensitive to bee stings he should be most strongly advised to give up keeping bees. He usually finds this advice very difficult to accept because a man may become as devoted to his bees as another man to his dog. It is often not until he has had his first anaphylactic reaction that he can be persuaded to give up keeping bees. Desensitization can be done but the risks of further reaction to a sting are still considerable.

Bird fancier's lung is a rare allergy and this type of allergy is dealt with more fully in Chapter 14 on Occupation and the Lung. It is a delayed type of sensitivity and is classified as a Type III allergy. It occurs rarely from the fungus in a budgerigar's or a pigeon's droppings and so can occur in pet owners. If it does occur the owner of the pet would be strongly advised to give up this particular interest so that the lung can heal up and no lasting damage be done.

There are a number of jobs which are connected with lung
disease. Of these probably the best known are pneu-
moconiosis connected with coal-miners, and asbestosis connected with workers with asbestos. Neither of these diseases, although they can be classified under occupation and
the lung, is an allergic disease. There are, however, a number
of allergic diseases of the lung connected with different occupations. Of these, the most common is farmer's lung.

Farmer's lung is due to a delayed type of hypersensitivity
which may be called more technically a Type III allergic
reaction to substances found in mouldy hay. It occurs in
many countries including the United Kingdom, Iceland and
the United States. In these countries the amount of the disease is closely connected with the amount of rainfall being
highest where the rainfall is highest. In the United Kingdom
there is most in the wetter parts of Scotland. The disease
was first described in 1932. It is now known as one of the
group of diseases called extrinsic allergic alveolitis.

The general cause of the trouble in farmer's lung is allergy
to the spores in mouldy hay. In parts of the country where

the rainfall is heavy the incidence can be as many as twenty times as high as that in drier parts of the country. In these areas the hay is often collected and stored while still wet. This is particularly likely to happen on small, ill-equipped farms where there are no drying or sileage facilities and often where the barns are not adequately ventilated. The damp hay heaped up gets very warm in the centre and this encourages the growth of fungus. When the farmer uses the stored hay as animal food during the winter, the mould is disturbed as the hay is tossed and minute particles of the dust are inhaled. It is particularly likely to happen in the winter months following an especially wet summer.

This type of extrinsic allergic alveolitis can happen in otherwise allergic and in otherwise normal people alike. There is no more often a family history of allergy than in the general population. Although it is called farmer's lung and it is generally assumed that it is a man that will be affected, it can also be the farmer's wife who gets the affliction. On small crofts in the north of Scotland the man often has an outside job to help ends meet financially and it is his wife and children who are left to tend the croft and feed the animals.

The farmer is not usually affected on his first exposure to mouldy hay because he has not developed the responsible antibodies. It may be many years before these antibodies develop. Once developed they react with the antigen in the mouldy hay when they come into contact with it. The group of substances which are responsible for producing the antigen and which are present in mouldy hay are the thermophilic actinomycetes. When the antigen and the antibodies meet in the lung a precipitate is formed and this does damage to the small blood vessels surrounding the alveoli. The alveoli are the tiny sacs right at the end of the smallest lung tubes through which normally the exchange of carbon dioxide and oxygen takes place.

The damage to the blood vessels sets up areas of inflammation in the lung which is sometimes called pneumonitis. An acute attack of farmer's lung occurs in a matter of hours, often about four, after exposure to the mouldy hay. It is very often not diagnosed during the first attack, but it is very important that doctors working among farmers in the affected areas of the United Kingdom should be ready to spot this illness. It is very important that it should be diagnosed, treated and further attacks prevented as quickly as possible. If repeated attacks are allowed to occur because the diagnosis is not made the victim can be left with permanent and considerable lung damage. When the chronic stage is reached there is little apart from the history of the illness to distinguish the condition from severe chronic bronchitis.

The patient usually does not start his illness until he is middle-aged. He is usually a farmer in a wet district, but can occasionally be a worker with animals who handles their food such as a zoo keeper. In the acute attack there are symptoms of a general illness and also of lung disease. The symptoms usually start between four and fifteen hours after exposure to mouldy hay. The patient feels very weak and has all the symptoms of a feverish illness. He has a headache, does not want to eat, feels and may be sick, and has aches and pains in his muscles. He is also very breathless and has a cough in which at first he brings up no sputum. He may have some wheezing, but usually breathing in is more difficult than breathing out, and in this way the illness is different from asthma, or other lung conditions which can be caused by mouldy hay. His temperature may be very high, the heart rate rapid and the breathlessness may be so severe as to make the patient turn a bluish tinge.

If the illness is not treated it lasts a few days and then the acute problems subside, but the feeling of weakness may last for several months. It is easy when the patient and doctor meet an acute illness like this to dismiss it as acute influenza or bronchitis, or acute asthma. It is important that the patient should be aware of the potential dangers of his occupation and that the doctor should know the type of diseases which he may meet in the area where he works, and be constantly on the look out for something such as farmer's lung.

The diagnosis can usually be clinched by the history of repeated exposure to possibly mouldy hay and by the number of hours delay between the last exposure and the start of this particular illness. It can usually be confirmed by laboratory tests for the presence of precipitating antibodies to the thermophylic actinomycetes in the blood. Chest X-ray is sometimes entirely normal at the first attack, but it may show a characteristic fine mottling which will help to make sure of the diagnosis.

It is very important that the diagnosis should be proved beyond doubt as soon as possible. The acute attack is then usually treated very successfully with steroids, tailing them off after four to six weeks. The vital part of treatment is to avoid further exposure to mouldy hay. If further exposure occurs there will certainly be more acute attacks of illness and eventually the chronic form will develop. In this the man is a semi-invalid unable to pursue any physically active job and with an entirely untreatable illness. The farmer who develops this illness is often not in a position financially to instal mechanical aids for drying and storing his hay or employing a man to handle his hay for him. It is often necessary to give up his occupation and doing this for a middle-aged man with no skill other than farming will not be advised light-heartedly. The fact remains that the only way to avoid the chronic phase of farmer's lung is to avoid exposure to mouldy hay. Wearing a mask may help a little but the particles that do the damage are very small and will pass through most masks. Desensitization has no effect.

There is another disease that farmers can get from mouldy hay and that is allergy to aspergillus fumigatus. This can easily be muddled with farmer's lung caused by thermophilic actinomycetes. The diagnosis can usually be made by growing the fungus aspergillus fumigatus from the plugs of mucus that the sufferer coughs up out of his lungs. It can also be made by a positive skin reaction to a prick test with a solution of aspergillus fumigatus. There is an immediate reaction showing a weal and flare and being characteristic of a Type I sort of sensitivity. There is also a delayed reaction occurring after about four hours which is characteristic of a Type III allergic reaction. In this illness there is a raised number of white blood cells, the eosinophils, both in the sputum and in the blood. In this type of lung disease there is no raised amount of the immunoglobulin IgE in the blood. In farmer's lung caused by thermophilic actinomycetes there is a raised amount of the immunoglobulin IgE, but not IgG.

The treatment of asthma in farmers caused by allergy to aspergillus fumigatus is principally to avoid exposure to the fungus. In its acute stages the illness can usually be helped by a short course of steroids. The result using bronchodilatators is poor. A similar type of asthma as that caused by aspergillus fumigatus can occur in workers manufacturing non-soap washing powders. This is an allergy to the enzymes produced from bacterial breakdown in the manufacturing process. This can be diagnosed in a similar way to the previous disease. Once this type of asthma has developed it will usually be necessary for the sufferer to change his job.

Allergic asthma with an immediate and delayed type of skin reaction can happen in a great number of occupations. These include working with platinum salts, producing antibiotics including ampicillin, workers with plastics including polyurethane products and some bleaches used by hairdressers. Some of these if mild may be prevented by the regular use of Intal but if severe a change of occupation will be necessary. Millers are also at risk of this trouble if they become allergic to inhaled flour.

There are other types of extrinsic allergic alveolitis seen besides farmer's lung. One of these is bird breeder's lung, or bird fancier's lung, and occurs as a result of close contact with the droppings of birds. It can rarely occur as the result of keeping a pet budgerigar. It is rare but must be thought of when somebody who has been in close contact with even one bird develops an obscure illness with chesty and general symptoms. A more common form of this disease is known as Byssinosis, and occurs in workers with cotton most often but also flax, and occasionally workers with soft hemp fibre. The disease was first described a very long time ago in 1832. The first signs of the disease are a feeling of tightness in the chest coming on some hours after starting work on the first day of work after a break. This is mostly common on a Monday after a weekend at home.

It usually takes ten years or more of working with cotton

or flax for symptoms to start to appear. It may be a general tiredness before the recurrent chest tightness starts. It occurs in various parts of the world where cotton is milled, including Lancashire, India, the United States and Egypt. The early part of the process in the carding rooms gives off most dust and it is the workers at this job who are at greatest risk. This condition is probably caused partly by the release of histamine in the lung tubes caused by the dust that is given off by the cotton.

Later in the disease there are attacks of wheezing and breathlessness. If tests of lung function are done at this stage the function is found to be severely impaired. Eventually the sufferer looks as though he has severe chronic bronchitis. At this stage the disease is permanent and very difficult to treat. The patient usually has to give up his work.

The diagnosis should be made as early as possible on the history of being in contact with a dusty process in the cotton or flax industry. When tiredness starts lung function tests should be done before waiting for further and irreversible trouble.

Prevention is difficult. Larger particles of dust can be removed from the working environment by extraction means, but the smaller particles which do the most harm to the lung are very difficult to remove. Increased mechanisation now means that fewer workers are left to do the dangerous jobs. Any man who shows early signs of trouble should be removed from work in a dusty atmosphere. Smokers are more at risk than non-smokers in developing this problem so there is yet one more reason why smoking should be abandoned.

15 Allergy and the mind

❖❖❖❖

Perhaps a better title for this chapter would be allergy and emotion. Whatever word is used to connect the mind or emotion and the body, it must be realised in this chapter all the time that it is not conscious will that is being discussed but the subtle and subconscious connection between mind and body. There is no place here for such words and phrases as 'fault', 'all in the mind', or 'pulling yourself together'. The connections that exist are quite different from this, and an entirely different attitude is necessary on the part of the doctor and the patient.

In medical terms there is a group of illnesses that is called psychosomatic. After the last world war there was a vogue for discussing and diagnosing this group of illnesses. They included such widely diverse problems as asthma, stomach ulcers, ulcerative colitis, or inflammation of the large bowel. There was a tendency amongst both doctors and patients once a diagnosis of psychosomatic illness had been made to undervalue the physical part of the illness. The patient could be left with the feeling that he was in some way responsible for his illness and easily become demoralised.

The present trend is in the opposite direction but there is still the split between physical and emotional causes. The truth is probably that there is no division between mind and body. The split exists only in the thinking of the doctor and the patient of the division between the mind and the body. The term psychosomatic now is used in an attempt to treat the patient as a whole and his illness as an integral part of the whole person. The physical entity of the brain and the nervous system and the less obviously concrete parts of the emotions and hormones are completely interdependent. Butterflies in the stomach are known to most of us and it is not necessary to see butterflies in the peritoneal cavity to know that the feeling may stem from fear or pre-examination nerves.

Basically in primitive man a state of fear produced by emotions and mind on the body would have prepared the individual to either fight or flee. This is no longer the generally accepted pattern in our civilisation. It is still accepted by the less inhibited, and occasionally the adolescent especially under the influence of alcohol. In the majority of people, however, a process of social conditioning takes place from the time of birth on that certain forms of behaviour are acceptable and that others are not acceptable. Over the years these norms change but some patterns remain even in the most permissive society. Time was when it was not acceptable for a baby to cry for food in less than the magic time of four hours. The pendulum swung and the baby was fed on demand. It was some years before the penny dropped that the baby might cry for other reasons than hunger and that the mother had some rights as well as the baby.

It is very difficult for members of the medical profession to treat each person seen as an individual with a unique personality, a unique illness, and unique problems. In training the medical student, emphasis is put on diagnostic labels and in later training a specialty must be selected. General medicine is split off from psychiatry which does nothing to help the treatment of the patient as a unique whole. It is the general practitioner who is in the best position to see the uniqueness and the wholeness of each of his patients. He may know his patient in health as well as in sickness, and with any luck knows a bit or a lot about his family and his job.

In allergic illnesses probably more than in any other type of illness there must be an interplay between the physical illness and the thoughts and emotions of the sufferer. This is partly because allergic illnesses are often long-standing ones and ones that have to be lived with instead of operated on or cured with an antibiotic. There is also emotional and mental interplay because of the effects of some allergic illnesses. Asthma is an extremely frightening illness both for the patient and for his relatives and friends. Fighting for breath can be like fighting for life itself and although very unlikely there is always the remote possibility that the patient could die during a severe and prolonged attack known as status asthmaticus. This has been discussed more fully in Chapter 4 on Asthma.

A sudden state of fear can have a profound effect on the physical functioning of the body. The skin can go white and cold, the eyes can dilate, the patient may vomit or have diarrhoea. He may shake. As has been said above in the primitive state he would fight or run. A chronic state of anxiety or tension may have an even more profound effect on the body however. In this civilisation the chronic state including a chronic state of frustration is more likely than an acute attack of fear. The patient may be doing a job he does not like, but cannot give up because of the mortgage payments on his house to be kept up. He may be working with people with whom he does not get on well. There may be marital problems at home, or difficulties with adolescent children. There are any number of stressful situations with which any of us may have to live.

So why is it that we don't all develop psychosomatic illness of one sort or another? There are a number of possibilities. In allergic illnesses one of these is genetic. In at least half of the people with allergy there is a family history of allergy which is far more than would be accounted for by the general incidence of 10% in the population. It is possible that in people with a hereditary predisposition to some illness it may take less to trigger off the illness whatever the cause may be, an allergen or an emotional upheaval. There is another line of thought that suggests in some people one system of the body may have a certain weakness. For example the gut may be at a disadvantage or the circulatory system. The third possibility why we do not all have psychosomatic illnesses is that some people can deal with tension and frustration better than others.

Attempts have been made to draw a profile of the sort of person liable to develop an allergic illness. There is no convincing evidence that in general, people with allergic diseases are more neurotic than those without. Some patients are believed to be very particular or obsessional people. They may be very conscientious and possibly overanxious. Perhaps the significant factor is that they tend to be people who bottle up their resentments and aggressive feelings. Although many normal and highly successful people may be overanxious and obsessional it is possible that the important factor in the production of allergic illness is the inability to show aggressive or hostile feelings. There is no proof, but it is certainly possible that the inability to show hostile feelings may be a common factor in people suffering from allergy.

The more civilised we become the less acceptable it is to show our real feelings. Temper tantrums at two may be acceptable but a blazing rage at forty is a very different matter and has to be kept under control perhaps precipitating an attack of asthma in the process of control. It is not proven, but certainly it is a possibility.

It is important at this point to say that if you have an allergy and know that you have problems, it is important that you should not start soul-searching or some form of self-analysis on your own. Problems should always be aired in the company of somebody else in whom you have complete trust and who will for preference take a neutral but constructive attitude. Very often it will be your general practitioner who can play such a role.

There is certainly a reciprocal action between allergy and emotion. Allergy of various sorts can most surely provoke emotional responses. During the hay fever season it may be noticed that the sufferer who may be normally equable becomes moody, tense, depressed and irritable. This may be partly because of disturbed nights and the constant discomfort. Long-standing skin disorders such as widespread eczema can lead to profound depression. The patient may feel that the whole world has a feeling of distaste for him because of the look of his skin. The constant itching is exhausting and the doctor, if he has not been successful in treating the condition may add to the patient's depression by showing his loss of patience and of confidence in his curative ability. Asthma can produce grave anxiety in the patient or in the instance of a child in the child's parents. This is entirely natural and normal.

There is another possibility. The allergy and the emotional upset may occur together but both be due to another cause. Hay fever may coincide with anxiety in the hay fever season because it is also the time when many public examinations are taken. Both the allergy and the emotional upset are due to coincidental factors and are only indirectly related to each other.

When you first see a doctor about an allergic illness he will make an investigation as described in Chapter 2. When he is taking the detailed history which is described fully in that chapter, he will probably enquire about any emotional factors which seem to act as triggers to allergic episodes or more long-standing emotional problems. Some people do seem to react easily to emotional upsets or feelings. Aroused sexual feelings can be accompanied by an attack of allergic rhinitis. The same people who are easily affected by emotional changes may also be affected by changes in temperature, or humidity, a slight cold or sore throat. The patient may know that worry or anger can bring on an attack of asthma.

It is very important that the doctor should not look for emotional causes to the exclusion of allergic ones. Allergic ones can be very much more easily dealt with. A course of desensitizing injections to the house dust mite where applicable may be very much more effective than probing of the psyche although there may be a great deal of emotional upset going hand in hand with the asthma. Particularly in children when the parents are naturally anxious and protective it is all too easy for a doctor to label them as over-anxious and overprotective and make them feel very guilty and personally responsible for their child's illness. It may be taken as a sign of emotional cause for the asthma when the child improves on removal to a boarding school. This is a possible factor but it is also possible that he has been removed from the house dust mite or family pet, to which he may be sensitive in his own home. It is an unwise doctor who concentrates on emotional factors to the exclusion of allergic or infective ones. The patient will naturally feel resentment towards his doctor if the latter has delved into emotional problems and missed out on allergic ones.

On the other hand the doctor must always be ready to accept the emotional problems of his patient as part of that patient's entire make-up. The patient too must be prepared to discuss his problems if he really wants his doctor to be able to help him as a whole and unique person. If you do not trust your doctor, or feel that you have lost confidence in him, or feel that you cannot discuss anything with him, you should think very hard. It is always difficult to change a doctor especially one to whom one has gone for a considerable time, but trust is an essential in any form of treatment. This applies very much to an allergic illness because there will be repeated visits to your doctor if the allergy is at all severe. Going to a specialist really does not solve the problem. If you attend repeatedly at a hospital out-patients the chances are that you will not always see the same doctor. If you see a specialist privately he will probably advise on your diagnosis and treatment and then send you back to your own doctor.

If there are severe emotional problems or a depressive illness which might be the result of an allergic problem or a coincidental one, it may be necessary to see a psychiatrist. By and large this is seldom necessary and your family doctor is by far the best person for help of all kinds including emotional problems. Hence the need for trust and the ability to be able to cooperate with him in your treatment.

All doctors are busy but the wise doctor will find time to listen to your history both of allergic illness and any other problems. It is perhaps especially necessary that a doctor should find time to listen to a patient who is also a mother. On a mother's health depends the well-being of her whole family. Most men can take time off work and be looked after without anything too drastic happening to the family, unless the illness is very long-standing or incapacitating. A mother cannot do this because not many mothers have anybody who can take over the house if they are laid up. Not many men can take time off work if their wives are ill. On the calm, patience and cheerfulness of the wife and mother, the well-being of the entire family depends. Husbands and fathers are less likely to become depressed in the early and middle years because they have two spheres of life at home and at work. Although many men find it difficult to discuss their problems they can still act out their problems occurring in one sphere in the other sphere and so obtain relief. A wife and mother has no such safety valve. She may confide in a friend but often the advice received is sympathetic rather than constructive. Many women become very lonely and depressed as housewives and the addition of an allergic illness naturally does nothing to help their gloom. It is very important indeed that such a woman should be able to unburden herself to a doctor.

Most patients' problems can be helped by a general practitioner even though he has had no specialised training in psychiatry. The patient knows that the discussion will be confidential. He must feel that his doctor will accept him just as he is with possibly a skin disease and a marital problem as well. He must also feel sure that the doctor will be sympathetic and will in no way pass judgement on him. He will need understanding, support and reassurance for a start.

There are basically two sorts of problems with which the patient and his doctor will have to cope. The first is the problem about which something can be done and the second is the problem about which nothing can be done. The first sort of problem may need action of one sort or another. There may be a marital problem which could be helped either by a doctor or by referral to a marriage guidance counsellor. There may be severe tensions at work in which case the patient might think about changing his job. The employment exchange could be a help or vocational guidance and retraining might be necessary. There may be financial worries where the advice of a good accountant could be more beneficial than any amount of antihistamines or tranquillisers.

The second type of problem is that about which nothing can be done. This sort of problem can occur in a mother with young children whose allergic problems are always worse before her period. It will help her if she realises that this is so, and it may help if she has appropriate treatment for her allergy, or her tension. Basically, however, the greatest help comes from realising that the condition occurs to her in this way and that she is in no way responsible for the internal supply of her hormones. There are many problems about which nothing at all can be done. Changing the environment has often been tried but it is usually without any long-lasting success. Such changes are often suggested because the doctor feels that he has failed in treating an illness so he must do something positive. Boarding school is suggested for a child, or moving house, or changing occupation.

It is possible that such a move will do good but if there is no scientific reason for the change the chances are there will be no lasting improvement in the allergic condition. The most important thing of all may be that the patient should change his attitude to his problems. The patient may already know that when he is calm and relaxed he has no allergic problems but when he lives under stress of one sort or another he is much more likely to have asthma or urticaria or whichever allergy it is to which he is prone. It has been said before that a psychological characteristic often found in people with allergies is an inability to let go and express aggressive feelings. A sympathetic doctor may be able to help his patient through this hurdle so that he can see what his suppressed emotions may be doing to him. Even if he does not change his boss or his wife, he may be able to change his attitude to one of these or anybody else who may be in part responsible for his illness. This does not mean that he has to go and have a blazing row with anybody but rather that he may be helped in admitting in the company of a sympathetic doctor that these problems exist, and then in the future he may be able to help himself a great deal.

If the patient is very tense and anxious it may help him generally and his allergy in particular, if he takes sedatives or tranquillisers for a while, and his doctor will advise him on this and recommend them if he feels they are necessary. In middle-aged and elderly people especially, it may be necessary to use antidepressant drugs if there is much depression. If depression becomes very severe whether connected with the allergy or coincidental your doctor will probably advise a visit to a psychiatrist.

Sympathy, support and understanding mean much more on the part of the doctor than a touch of bedside manner and a pat on the back. Time, patience and a real understanding of the patient and his problems are necessary if a doctor is going to be able to give really effective and lasting help.

16 Holidays and allergy

❖❖❖

When leaving the United Kingdom for a holiday it is always a good idea to make plans for health care while abroad. This is especially important if you have any form of allergy because at best it is usually a chronic or recurrent illness, and at worst an entirely new environment. You may well come across something that will make the allergy flare up. In some countries in Europe, including the common market countries, there are arrangements for us to have free medical treatment under the insurance schemes. Application must be made for this exchange type of insurance on form CM1 which is obtainable from your local social security office. You will be sent certificate E111 entitling you to treatment in these countries. It may take several weeks to receive this certificate, particularly in the holiday season, and therefore application should be made for it at least six weeks before your departure.

It is as well to check that any reciprocal arrangements exist with the country to which you are travelling. If there are none or you are travelling outside Europe it is wise to take out a private health insurance. This can usually be done through a travel agent or with the firm that handles your other insurance such as fire and life. It is important to remember that the costs of medical treatment are considerably higher in other countries than they are even in private medicine in the United Kingdom. It is as well to make the amount of insurance on the generous side because there is always the remote possibility of an acute appendicitis as well as a sharp attack of hay fever or other allergy.

This makes going on holiday sound a depressing affair for the allergic patient and certainly there are a number of problems that should be sorted out. This chapter is an attempt to help sort out some of those problems and so make a holiday more comfortable and illness free. Now that holidays are taken so much further afield you may run into a seasonal allergy at quite an unexpected time. The hay fever season even in the north of Scotland is several weeks later than in the south of England. A holiday taken in Scotland after symptoms have just about cleared up in the south may well provoke a further attack. I had my worst ever attack of hay fever last year at the end of November. That was in Melbourne, Australia. It took me several days to realise what had hit me and of course I had gone unprepared without any antihistamine tablets.

If you are on any tablets or medicine for an allergy it is a good idea to see your own doctor before you leave and get an adequate supply of your necessary medicine. It may even be necessary to get extra if you are going to the country and have hay fever or pollen asthma. In any case it is a good idea to have a brief discussion with your doctor before your holiday about necessary medicines and other precautions. Buying tablets or medicines abroad can be an extremely expensive business. It may on the other hand be possible to buy the drugs freely over the counter of a chemist's shop because in many countries, especially outside Europe, the regulations for drug prescription are not as tight as in the United Kingdom. If you have to buy drugs abroad it is useful if you know the actual name of the drug in your particular tablet or medicine. Trade names may vary from country to country but it will be possible probably to get a drug with the same active ingredient. If the name of the basic drug is not on your tin or bottle, it is as well to ask your doctor and then note it down in your diary or other notebook that you are sure to be taking away with you. Bits of paper for this purpose are a menace because they always turn up in the wrong pocket or handbag.

Hay fever can be one of the worst holiday hazards to cope with. It is important to remember the hay fever season in the country to which one is going. If this is the other side of the world it may be advisable to have a course of desensitizing injections after the end of the season in the United Kingdom. If hay fever is at all severe, and especially if pollen asthma starts, it is probably necessary to have a course of desensitizing injections but your doctor will decide this. In the south of England it is better not to have a holiday in the country in June or July. Camping is probably better avoided at any time for those who are likely to get severe hay fever. Although a course of desensitizing injections is often relatively successful it will not protect a person against exposure to very large doses of grass pollen or to whichever pollen you are sensitive.

High altitudes are better for holidays than sea level and the Swiss Alps are often very suitable. If it were not for the unfavourable rate of exchange this might be acceptable to more sufferers. A long sea voyage is also good but often there is the problem of cost especially when a whole family's holiday is involved. If it is impossible to avoid exposure to pollen it will be as well to discuss the problem with your doctor especially if you have not already had a course of desensitizing injections. He may suggest taking antihistamines or disodium cromoglycate as a nasal application. Again with antihistamines they should be tried out before the holiday and you must never start on a long car journey before knowing the effects on you if you are driving. It is also important with all sports, especially such ones as hill climbing or water skiing where awareness and balance are particularly important to know the effect of the antihistamine before indulging in the sport. Any unaccustomed activity is specially important to try out under safe conditions while taking an antihistamine. Some doctors are prepared to give an injection of a longacting steroid immediately before going on a holiday. This will last for anything from two to four weeks. It is not done to demand any particular treatment from your doctor and you will have to discuss the particular problem with him and he will prescribe the treatment he considers most effective for you.

When travelling in the hay fever season it is better to keep car and train windows shut. In a train you have less control because there may be a fresh air fiend or two in the same compartment. For this reason travelling by car especially through country areas may be preferable. If you are absolutely obliged to camp, or cannot resist it, fine wet muslin should be clipped over your tent ventilators at night and the doors kept shut.

If you are taking antihistamine tablets regularly or for the first time on holiday it is important to remember that the effects of alcohol on top of the antihistamine may make you very drowsy. This is particularly important if you are taking antihistamine tablets for the first time. It is also more important if you are taking a holiday in a country where alcohol is cheaper especially wine and you are likely to have a higher intake of alcohol. At least do not drink, drive and take antihistamines until you are sure what the combined effect is.

Rynacrom or disodium cromoglycate for the nose if taken regularly may control the symptoms for the length of a holiday. Or possibly steroids taken as a snuff may be effective. If the hay fever is confined mostly to the eyes as an allergic conjunctivitis it may be effective to use corticosteroid eyedrops. These are quite safe if only used for a short time. It may also be helpful with allergic conjunctivitis to take antihistamines at night. Allergic conjunctivitis does not only occur as a reaction to grass pollen but can occur in response to other pollen or moulds. It is very likely to occur with a change in the allergens to which you are exposed and so is particularly likely to start on holiday. It may be impossible to be prepared for this and will very likely mean a visit to a doctor if it is at all troublesome.

Asthma may occur on holiday for several reasons. It may

be pollen asthma and part of hay fever. If this has occurred once it is a good reason for having desensitizing injections in the following year. It should always be taken seriously and medical help obtained if you are not already prepared for it and know which drugs and how much to take. Asthma may occur if you go and stay in an old cottage particularly in a warm damp place. These conditions encourage the growth of the house dust mite and being in close touch with an increased number of these menaces may well trigger off asthma particularly at night. If you know you are allergic to the house dust mite it is often worth having one of the short courses of desensitizing injections. If the allergy takes you unawares it would probably be a good idea to have it fully investigated on your return. If you are returning to the same cottage the next year a course of desensitizing injections may be indicated if the house dust mite or a mould was found to be responsible for the trouble.

If you know you are sensitive to the house dust mite and are already sleeping on a rubber mattress and pillows another problem arises. It is not usually possible to take all ones bedroom equipment on holiday because of the space problem. It is well worth taking a very large sheet of polythene for covering the new mattress and large polythene bags for covering the pillows. A roll of Sellotape will help you to seal in the mites effectively. This is just one more thing to remember when going on holiday but may make all the difference between a lovely healthgiving rest and a miserable wheezing fortnight.

There are several skin hazards which are particularly likely to occur on holiday. One of these is urticaria which is described more fully in Chapter 9 on Urticaria. Especially on the continent we are more likely to eat fish as a meal in a sauce or a snack. Fish is one of the most likely causes of food induced urticaria. Oysters and mussels and many other fish may be responsible. Children eating some fish or fruit for the first time may come out in an urticarial rash. Usually the urticaria subsides quite quickly and if a particular food is suspected it should be avoided. Calamine put on the skin helps the itchiness and it may be necessary to get some antihistamines to take at night if you have not already got a supply.

Rarely a condition called cold urticaria can occur and this also is described in Chapter 9 on Urticaria. It may run in the family or may start at any age. Urticarial weals come up on any part of the body exposed to chilling which may be either low temperature in the air, chill winds or cold water. Anybody with this condition should be warned about the dangers of swimming in cold water. Occasionally the throat may swell while drinking an iced drink. Extreme chilling can cause a state of anaphylactic shock and collapse. The kiss of life may be necessary if the person stops breathing and medical help should be got as fast as possible.

The kiss of life or mouth to mouth resuscitation is considered to be the most effective form of artificial respiration. Anybody can do it by just reading how, and without any practical instruction. It should be done on anybody who has stopped breathing and in this context it is a useful thing to know about on holiday for other casualties besides allergic ones. Speed is all important and one minute can make all the difference between success and failure. The casualty should be rolled on to his back and his mouth quickly cleared of mucus or false teeth. One hand should be put under the back of his neck and lifted so that the chin comes up and forwards. Take a deep breath in and if it is an adult hold his nose and opening your mouth put it firmly against the margins of his and breathe out firmly until you see his chest rise. Then take your head away, turn it to one side and take in a deep breath. This should be repeated about ten times a minute. If it is a child you should put your open mouth over his nose and mouth and breathe out much more gently until you see his chest rise. This should be done about fifteen to twenty times a minute, depending on the age of the child. You should continue with the kiss of life until medical help or the ambulance with trained helpers arrives.

Exposure to sun can cause skin problems in some people. Sometimes it occurs when a person is taking a drug such as sulphonamides, some tranquillisers and occasionally the contraceptive pill. A very short time in the sun can cause a rash on the exposed parts. Sometimes it can be caused by antibacterial substances in soap or cream that is used on the skin. Antihistamines used on the skin in creams or lotions can cause serious trouble especially on exposure to the sun. Antihistamines should never be used on the skin and although freely available in chemists' shops should not be used in combination with calamine lotion or cream. It is possible to get sun barrier creams and your doctor or chemist will advise you on a suitable one.

Insect bites and stings can be very troublesome to somebody who has been sensitized to them. Bee and wasp stings can be really dangerous in the sensitized person. In the United States these insects cause more deaths than any other venomous animal and in addition many near fatalities. When first stung by an insect there is not usually any serious reaction. There may however be considerable swelling and redness at the site of the sting. There may also be a spreading urticaria surrounding the bite and occasionally there are more general reactions. These can include shivering, sneezing or wheezing. If these things happen after a wasp or bee sting you should see your doctor. Stings from other insects seldom cause a general reaction although they can cause troublesome local reactions. These are a nuisance rather than a danger.

Insect bites are best avoided by those who are allergic to them. Ordinary midge bites can best be avoided by keeping away from midge ridden areas. This includes fishing in the summer months in Scotland. Wearing protective clothing including trousers and thin ankle socks helps. It is possible to get anti-midge creams and sprays but these only give partial protection and for a short time. All chemists sell these creams and it is worth using them on exposed parts such as the face. It is worth using a midge killing repellant in the house where you are staying and particularly in the bedroom before you undress. The best treatment for midge bites is calamine used on the skin and antihistamine preparation taken at night if necessary.

Bee and wasp stings once having produced any general reaction should be taken seriously. One general reaction is usually taken as a good reason for a course of densensitizing injections. These may not give complete protection but usually save the sufferer from any severe or fatal reaction. The real danger is anaphylactic shock in the sensitized person leading to collapse and even death. Bees are not very likely to sting if left to themselves. Wasps are far more vicious and should be avoided by anybody known to be sensitive to their stings. If a wasps' nest is known in the United Kingdom the local sanitary department will provide somebody to dispose of it for a modest fee. Orchards where there are rotting fruit should always be avoided. If wasps appear during the course of a picnic the allergic person should hop quickly into the car or indoors and shut the windows.

The person who has had a severe reaction from a bee or wasp sting may be given an emergency kit by his doctor. This will probably be a syringe with adrenalin and the patient will be given instructions for its use. This can be life saving. If somebody is allergic to a sting and has one from a wasp there is nothing that can be done at the site of the sting. If it is from a bee the venom sac is left at the site of the sting and this should be removed. The most effective way of doing this without getting more venom into the patient's system is by flicking it out with the point of a sharp knife or penknife. The patient should be put flat on the ground and the stung arm or leg raised and supported in a raised position.

A tourniquet may be put round the limb on the heart side of the sting. A tourniquet may be made from a large handkerchief, or belt or a tie. It should be put on tight enough to make the veins stand out but not tight enough to stop the pulse at the wrist or the ankle. If a tourniquet is put on it should be loosened for a minute every quarter of an hour. The patient should be got to hospital or medical help obtained as quickly as possible. If the patient has other allergies such as asthma he may have isoprenaline tablets and one of these dissolved under the tongue will help the state of shock.

It is usual for most women and some men to buy new clothes before going on a holiday. If you are allergic in any way it is a good idea to try these clothes out before taking them away. Synthetic underwear can cause a rash and so can the dyes in some materials if brought out by perspiration. This can also happen in the dyes in some shoes. If in any doubt forget about being trendy and stick to well-tried clothes that have never caused you any trouble. New cosmetics bought for the holiday may also in combination with heat produce rashes or allergic conjunctivitis. Again it is best to try them out on hot days before the holiday and if in doubt leave them behind. It is not worth wearing beautiful new eye shadow if it wrecks your holiday with streaming eyes.

One last point to remember is that if you or any member of your family is allergic it is important to tell any doctor who treats you during the holiday even if it is not for an illness that is an allergic one. The two most important sensitivities to remember and to report are allergy to penicillin and allergy to aspirin. These allergies will obviously not be known to a strange doctor, and they will affect the treatment he will prescribe for an illness.

If you remember that allergies can always crop up however healthy you should be you will learn to live more peaceably with them and this applies especially to holiday times.

17 Auto-immunity and allergy

❖❖❖

Work on auto-immunity or auto-allergy as it is now sometimes called is still very much in the experimental stage. It involves so many ideas and so many illnesses and so much research that it is difficult to give practical advice to possible sufferers. It is however included here because there is now good evidence that it involves an allergic type of reaction and probably with further research it will be found that quite common illnesses will come under the classification of auto-immune diseases.

At present the whole range of fairly well established auto-immune diseases covers such a wide variety of diseases as one sort of thyroid disease, rheumatoid arthritis and more than one sort of anaemia. Current research is all the time opening up quite extraordinary new posibilities and there has been an idea that some sorts of mental illness could be forms of auto-immunity. This, it must be emphasised, implies only an idea and much research needs to be done.

Normally in an allergic reaction the body produces its allergy to what may be called a 'foreign' protein. Not all allergens are proteins but a great many of them are. In auto-immunity the general idea is that the body turns its hostility against its own 'self' proteins and so tries to destroy itself. This might be called civil war between its various parts, or even a suicidal type of reaction on the part of the body. The way in which the body normally distinguishes 'foreign' antigens from 'self' antigens is still not fully understood. However in auto-immune diseases there is a failure to recognise 'self' antigens and the whole allergic mechanism is turned by the body against itself.

Probably what happens in auto-immune diseases is something like this but there are still so many unknowns and work on these diseases is still in its early stages. Some unknown cause produces damage of a body tissue. Particles of this damaged tissue are then released into the body and the particles do not have the same characteristics as the normal tissue. The particles then act as antigens or allergens and trigger off an allergic response. The response triggered is shown to be an allergic one and there is a typical antigen antibody sort of response with a precipitate formed. There may be a vicious circle built up where damage of the tissues causes an allergic reaction with release of antigens which in its turn produces precipitate which produces further damage of the organ and so on.

It is thought that this type of disease may run in families and that members of these families are more likely through inheritance to have the sort of failure in recognition of their own tissues that happens in this group of diseases. In some diseases for example rheumatoid arthritis, what is called a precipitating antibody specific for this disease may be found in the patient's blood if it is examined. It is very interesting that in the patient's close relations the same precipitating antibody may be found in their blood streams. Although people with the increased amount of precipitating antibody in their blood may not at the time of examination show any signs of rheumatoid arthritis they are more likely to develop it in later years.

Two main groups of auto-immune disease have been described. In the first group only one organ or one system of the body is affected. In the second group several organs or systems of the body may be affected.

Of the first group a good example in Hashimoto's thyroiditis. This sounds a very imposing name and it is an extremely interesting condition. It is probably the best understood of all the auto-immune diseases. At first the thyroid gland enlarges. This causes swelling in the front of the neck that moves up and down on swallowing. The patient usually goes to his or her doctor at first to complain about the swelling. The enlarged thyroid is firm to feel and has clearly demarcated edges. If blood tests are done on such a patient it will be found that there are precipitating antibodies present to his own thyroid tissue. In other words his thyroid has started acting to his body as though it were an outside or foreign allergen and antibodies are produced against it. If blood tests are done on close relatives of the patient it will be found that some of them also have precipitating antibodies to thyroid gland.

If nothing is done about this type of thyroid enlargement or goitre eventually the antibodies will kill off the whole of the thyroid gland. The swelling in the neck will get smaller and harder, and eventually there will be no thyroid at all to feel or possibly a small fibrous lump will remain in place of the once active thyroid. The extracts of the thyroid gland which are vital for the body's proper functioning will gradually get less and will eventually disappear. During this process the patient will gradually show signs of deficiency of thyroid extract and eventually will show a complete picture of deficiency or as it is called medically myxoedema.

In myxoedema the patient is characteristically slowed down both physically and mentally. He, or more often she, will put on weight which is of course not unusual at any age, and is only rarely due to disease of the thyroid gland. She will feel the cold very much and prefer hot weather and heated rooms. One of the most marked signs is the progressive loss of hair which is particularly noticeable in a woman. Baldness may be a sign and loss of body hair. The outer third of the eyebrows may fall out. At this stage treatment is absolutely essential.

If the disease is caught in its early stages and treatment is started with the right amount of thyroxin the thyroid may soften up and become a more normal size. If, however, the disease is not diagnosed until a late stage thyroxin will have no effect on either the size or the texture of the thyroid gland. The doctor should make it plain to his patient when treating this disease that there is no actual cure but that replacement of the deficient or missing substance from the thyroid gland can maintain health for many years. It must be made clear to the patient that she is not taking drugs but a substance that is absolutely vital for her body's needs and which is deficient or lacking naturally because of the disease that has attacked her. She will need to take the thyroxin in sufficient doses for the rest of her life.

Another disease which is characteristic of the first group of auto-immune diseases in which only one organ or system of the body is involved is haemolytic anaemia. In this illness the patient turns on his own red cells in the blood and makes antibodies against them. Red blood cells are produced mainly in the marrow of bones and a normal red blood cell lives for about a hundred days. However one that has been attacked lives for only a few days. The marrow keeps working as hard as it can but it just cannot keep up with this enormously increased turnover of cells. The red blood cells are destroyed in the spleen which is an organ in the abdominal cavity, up under the left side of the rib cage. The spleen becomes much enlarged. Some of the pigment from the rapid destruction of red cells may make the patient jaundiced or yellow. The diagnosis can usually be made by finding the anaemia and increased size of the spleen. The diagnosis can be clinched by delicate laboratory tests in which it is found that the outside of the red blood cells are coated with antibody.

Again, as with Hashimoto's thyroiditis, there is no real cure. Health can usually be maintained by giving an immediate transfusion with blood to counteract the anaemia. It is no good leaving the matter at that because the new blood cells will be destroyed in the same way as the ones made in the patient's body. The next step is the removal of the spleen to slow up the breakdown of the red blood cells.

A further example of the first group of auto-immune diseases is pernicious anaemia. In this disease there is destruction of certain specialised cells in the lining of the stomach that affects the absorption of various vitamins including Vitamin B_{12}. Vitamin B_{12} is a vital ingredient for the formation of blood. The lining of the stomach becomes gradually more inflamed and eventually there is complete destruction of the special cells and no Vitamin B_{12} is absorbed at all. This causes pernicious anaemia. Nothing can be done to reverse the changes in the stomach or make the body capable of absorbing Vitamin B_{12} again in the normal way. The vital ingredient of blood can however be replaced by regular injections. Again as in the case of other auto-immune diseases already described nothing can be done to actually cure the disease but regular replacement can help the patient to remain in good health for many years.

The second group of diseases includes a disease called systemic lupus erythematosis or S.L.E. for short in which many parts of the body may be affected. These can include the joints, the skin, the spleen, the liver, kidneys and lung. Destruction of the kidneys is usually amongst the most severe damage done in this disease. The disease in some ways is like serum sickness, but in serum sickness as in other allergies previously described there is a spontaneous cure even if the condition is not treated. In S.L.E. there is no such cure and the destruction continues indefinitely. Again there is no real cure but the use of steroids can damp down the damage and prolong life and health.

Rheumatoid arthritis is another disease which probably comes in this group. Although the damage done is mostly to the linings of joints causing inflammation, pain and swelling, it can also sometimes affect the lungs and other parts of the body. Again although the self destruction of the body cannot yet be stopped, treatment especially with steroids can damp down the body's reaction and help the symptoms of the disease and its progressive destruction of the body's joints.

It is just possible that diabetes is sometimes an auto-immune disease in which the body destroys the insulin-producing cells in the pancreas. In some cases of untreated diabetes anti-insulin antibodies have been found in the blood. In the treatment of diabetes again it has to be said that there is no real cure but life and health can be prolonged by the regular taking of insulin or other drugs.

It is possible that in some way there is an emotional factor in all auto-immune diseases. It is possible that there is a hereditary tendency to develop an auto-immune disease but it may need emotional stress to trigger off the start of the disease.

As all auto-immune diseases are long drawn out affairs and in the case of rheumatoid arthritis potentially crippling, it is particularly important that sufferers from one of these diseases should get all the help and comfort and support they need from their doctors.

Index